Ski Flex

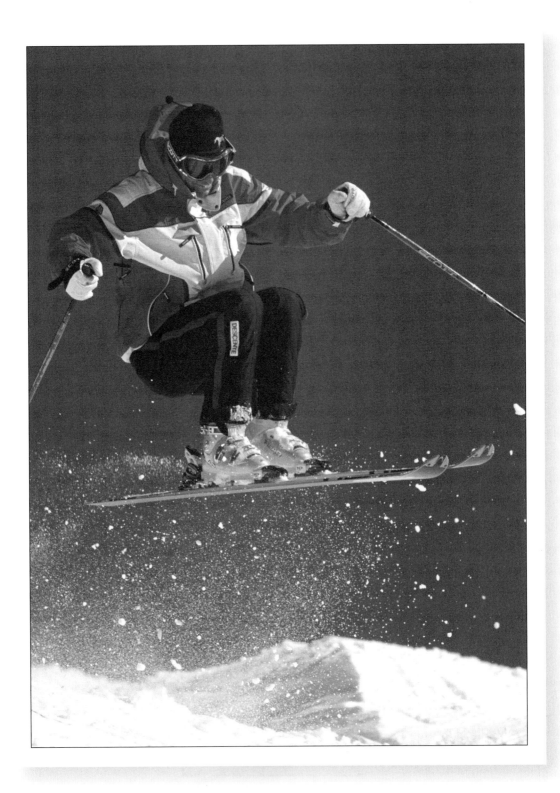

Ski Flex

Flexibility, Fitness
& Conditioning
for Better Skiing

Paul Frediani and Harald Harb

A Healthy Living Book
HATHERLEIGH PRESS
New York • London

Cover and interior design by Corin Hirsch
Photos by Jeff Cricco
Printed in Canada

Hatherleigh Press
An affiliate of W.W. Norton and Company, Inc.
5-22 46th Avenue, Suite 200
Long Island City, NY 11101

www.hatherleighpress.com

Library of Congress Cataloging-in-Publication Data

Frediani, Paul, 1952-
    Ski flex : better skiing through flexibility and conditioning / Paul Frediani and Harald Harb.
      p. cm.
    "A Healthy Living Book."
    ISBN 1-57826-058-2 (paper : alk. paper)
Skis and skiing—Training. 2. Stretching exercises. I. Harb, Harald R. II. Title.

GV854.85 .F74 2002
796.93—DC21

2002027516

10 9 8 7 6 5 4 3 2 1

For Skiers of All Abilities–
Everywhere.

Acknowledgments

I'd like to acknowledge my coauthor Harald Harb—one of skiing's leading authorities. Special thanks go also to my publisher and friend Andrew Flach.

—*Paul Frediani*

I would like to dedicate the book to Hermann Gollner. He had the greatest influence on me and inspired me to pursue a sports career.

—*Harald Harb*

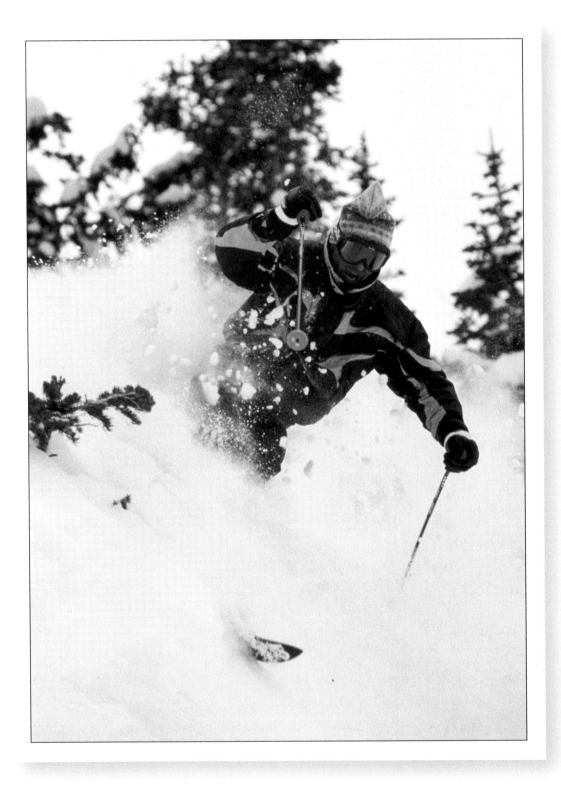

Contents

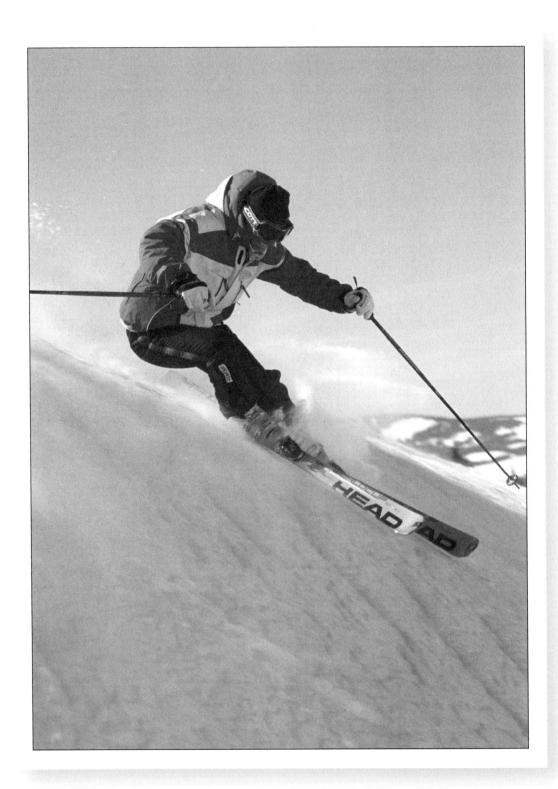

Introduction:
Welcome
to SkiFlex

YOU HAVE JUST TAKEN A POSITIVE STEP TO IMPROVE YOUR SKIING through proper flexibility and conditioning exercises.

Everyone from weekend warriors to professional athletes agree: They all dislike stretching. Why? Because they find it time-consuming, boring, and too complex.

Not anymore. Ski Flex is simple, quick, and enjoyable. Follow us and learn how flexibility can enhance your skiing experience in all terrain by helping you to move better and more efficiently—and to avoid the injuries that can be caused by poor movement. Think about it: You invest hundreds—even thousands—of dollars in ski equipment, lift tickets, transportation, and lodging for a ski vacation. Isn't it worth investing 10 or 15 minutes a day before you ski to ensure your safety and enjoyment? That's where Ski Flex comes in.

The Ski Flex program prepares and warms up the specific muscles you use on the mountain; that's called sports specificity. The program also encompasses functional stretching and explains how you can incorporate it into your everyday living activities. This is the essence of Ski Flex.

We're pretty sure that you didn't put on your skis for the first time and have a great day on the mountain. You developed the skill over time, training your muscles and learning to make them perform properly. The same holds true with stretching and flexibility: Consistency, plain and simple, is critical. If you move your body in specific motions, it will respond over a period of time. To improve your mobility, and thereby your skiing experience, you need to prepare the tendons, ligaments, and muscles that surround and support your joints in a similar manner. You won't achieve better range of motion in your joints unless you stretch regularly.

Ski Flex was developed not only to prepare you in a systematic and easy-to-follow way for your pre-ski warm-up, but also, very importantly, to help you find and create ways to add stretching to your life on a consistent basis. What more can you ask for than a program that is enjoyable and effective, yet not time-consuming?

Join us and discover a great new way to improve your skiing experience with the secrets of Ski Flex!

–Paul Frediani,
Personal Trainer

–Harald Harb,
Professional Skiing Consultant;
Trainer and Examiner of Ski Instructors;
Ski Racing, Master Coach, U.S. Ski Coaches Association

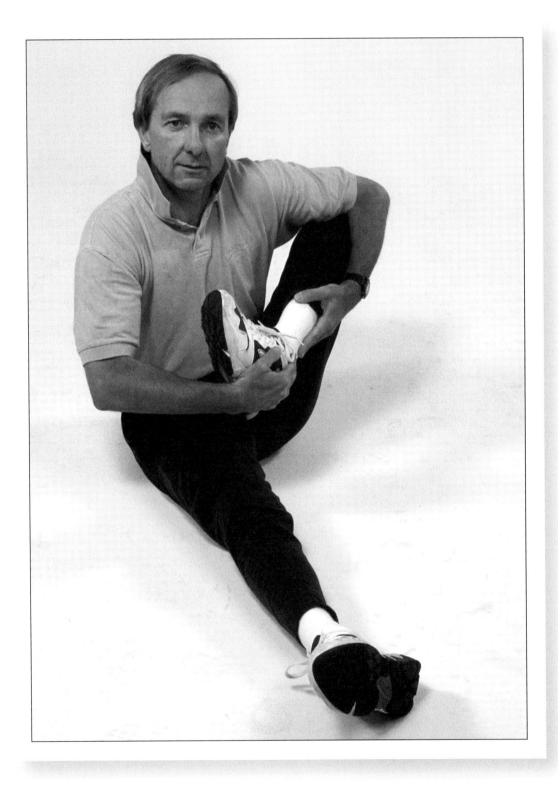

Part 1: **Why**
Stretch?
How Stretching
Prevents Injury

A PROPER WARM-UP AND STRETCH IS AN IMPORTANT PART OF PREPARING for a good day of skiing. You wouldn't get in your car on a cold day, start it up, and immediately race down the freeway at 60 miles per hour—your car wouldn't last you very long if you did. Your body is the most important piece of equipment you own, so you don't want to throw yourself down a mountain on two pieces of fiberglass, regardless of your skill, unless you know your body is ready to perform at the peak of its ability. Warming up and stretching are crucial to the process.

The American Academy of Orthopaedic Surgeons emphasizes that to keep your joints healthy, you must warm up and stretch. A good warm-up is necessary in part because it increases your body's core temperature by 1 to 2 degrees Celsius. According to the American College of Sports Medicine, "muscles at rest receive only 15 to 20 percent of blood pumped from the heart, but during vigorous exercise they may receive as much as 75 percent." So it is important to get the heart rate up properly and the blood flow to skeletal muscles. Warming up will also increase your body's coordination, reaction time, and accuracy of movement by engaging the neuromuscular system. It will increase the suppleness of connective tissues, making you less susceptible to musculotendinous injuries.

In 1998, 28,150 baby boomers—persons born between 1946 and 1964—were reported to have visited hospital emergency rooms with ski-related injuries. We'd bet that many of those injuries could have been prevented with a good warm-up and stretching program. Stretching can improve performance and decrease risk of injury by increasing the body's range of motion, improving muscular imbalances (a major cause of sports injuries), and helping to maintain good posture. It can also reduce soreness and the risk of lower back pain by increasing the flexibility of the hamstrings, quadriceps, and hip flexors. Stretching will also increase blood, nutrient, and synovial fluid flow to joints, which keeps the joints healthy by reducing wear and tear.

As we get older and become less active, we naturally lose flexibility, and this increases the risk of injury to our joints, tendons, and muscles. A consistent stretching program can reduce soreness and maximize your experience on the slopes—and it can even slow down the flexibility loss that comes with aging!

Aren't we all interested in maintaining independence in our lives through mobility? None of us want to be slaves to our injuries, which can become chronic and force us to give up our active lifestyles. With just a little effort and an awareness of our daily living habits, we can avoid most common skiing injuries. Many shoulder, back, knee, and hip injuries are a direct result of inflexibility, weak muscles, and poor postural habits. Thumb, calf, and/or head injuries are also common.

Stretching for Strength

Did you know that tightness is often a sign of muscular weakness? Flexibility and strength training go hand in hand. Identify your weakness and improve your strength. Conversely, did you know that stretching can also help strengthen weak muscles? True!

The Wrong Way to Stretch

Before we talk about the right way to stretch, let's discuss how *not* to stretch. After all, stretching the wrong way can be just as harmful as not stretching at all.

Stretching statically—stretching, holding it, and then moving to the next stretch—feels good, doesn't it? Yes, but save that slow stretching for a cool-down after your ski session, when it will reduce lactic acid in muscles, which can contribute to muscle soreness.

Another improper stretching method is called ballistic stretching. It's an active bouncing that uses the momentum of your body to force the joint to and from the end of its range of motion. Ballistic stretching is not considered useful and can actually lead to a tightening of the muscles. Proper stretching allows your muscles to gradually ease into a relaxed stretched position; ballistic stretching doesn't do that.

Before your ski run, you want your stretching to be active and dynamic. Stretching dynamically means moving in and out of stretch positions rhythmically and smoothly. Ski Flex uses dynamic stretching to prepare your muscles to move and react just as they do on the slopes, while raising your body temperature in preparation for that first run.

Stay with the Ski Flex program. Take just a little time each day to stretch and you'll be amazed at how quickly your body responds. Don't overstretch or give up if you miss a day. After a while, stretching will become as natural a part of your day as brushing your teeth.

The Benefits of Stretching

- Reduces risk of injury
- Increases range of motion
- Increases body awareness
- Improves circulation
- Reduces muscle tension
- Reduces soreness
- Relaxes and relieves stress

Stretching Isn't Always Enough . . .

Besides following the Ski Flex program, there are more steps you can take to improve your flexibility:

- Increase your awareness of day-to-day activities that can hurt you in the long run: sitting with your legs crossed, carrying a bag slung over your shoulder, working hunched over at your desk, and putting on ski boots before you're warmed up.

- Stand up straight. You can improve your flexibility by eliminating poor posture habits.

- Drink, drink, drink—water, that is. We lose flexibility as we get older

Myth-Information about Stretching

Here, once and for all, we dispel the myths you may have heard about stretching.

MYTH 1: IT'S TOO TIME-CONSUMING. There's no way I can fit it in my busy schedule. You don't need to take time out from your day to stretch. You can start a flexibility program before you even get out of bed, while working in the office, or even in the car. (See Part 3: Year-Round Conditioning, page 75.)

MYTH 2: FLEXIBILITY TRAINING IS FOR PROFESSIONAL ATHLETES ONLY. It is much too complex to do alone. I would have to hire a personal trainer and spend a fortune. Ski Flex is as easy as one, two, three. Complex fitness programs just don't work. If you have read this far, you're smart enough to follow this program. Save your money for a new pair of skis.

MYTH 3: I WILL NEVER BE FLEXIBLE. You will never be flexible if you don't stretch. You may never do splits, but you can significantly improve your range of motion. The aging process naturally shortens and tightens your muscles. Flexibility training can help reverse that process.

MYTH 4: I DON'T NEED TO STRETCH EVERYDAY. I stretch well just before I ski. Here's what stretching once a week will do for you: absolutely nothing. To increase your range of motion or improve flexibility, you need to stretch 10 minutes a day. Consistency is the key.

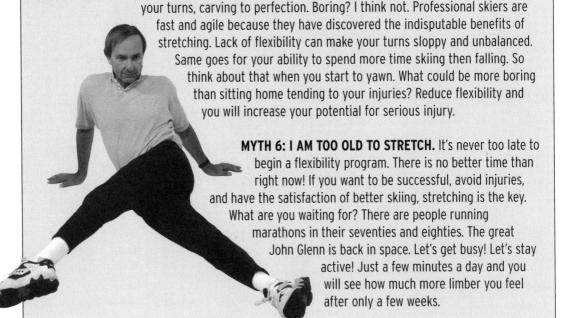

MYTH 5: STRETCHING IS SO BORING! Think about taking on more challenging terrain, speeding up your turns, carving to perfection. Boring? I think not. Professional skiers are fast and agile because they have discovered the indisputable benefits of stretching. Lack of flexibility can make your turns sloppy and unbalanced. Same goes for your ability to spend more time skiing then falling. So think about that when you start to yawn. What could be more boring than sitting home tending to your injuries? Reduce flexibility and you will increase your potential for serious injury.

MYTH 6: I AM TOO OLD TO STRETCH. It's never too late to begin a flexibility program. There is no better time than right now! If you want to be successful, avoid injuries, and have the satisfaction of better skiing, stretching is the key. What are you waiting for? There are people running marathons in their seventies and eighties. The great John Glenn is back in space. Let's get busy! Let's stay active! Just a few minutes a day and you will see how much more limber you feel after only a few weeks.

largely due to the lack of movement needed to transport fluids to our joints. Drinking plenty of water helps replenish these necessary fluids, thereby keeping our muscles flexible.

• Try to avoid caffeine and alcohol, or at least increase your water intake after drinking these beverages to reduce dehydration.

And remember, you can be very flexible in your lower body while still having a very tight upper body. The beauty of the Ski Flex program is that you can tailor it to address your body's individual flexibility needs.

The Skiing Environment

Skiing is an outdoor winter sport and that means skiers can encounter a wide range of weather conditions in a single day. What does this have to do with stretching? Those conditions can tighten your muscles, shorten your tendons, and sap your energy. Here are some of the factors you need to consider before you ski, and some ways to cope for a better day on the slopes.

Temperature and Precipitation

Our bodies perform much better and move more efficiently when they are warm and dry. And as any skier will tell you, getting—and staying—warm and dry is important for enjoyable skiing. Layering garments made of lightweight materials will provide excellent results. Many modern high-tech fabrics used for outerwear provide wind and moisture protection with breathability, which allows the body to shed accumulated moisture. Here's how to protect yourself— from head to toe.

• **Head.** Without a hat, you lose body heat quickly through the top of your head, and so a cold head means a cold body. A wool hat with a fleece liner or a 100-percent fleece hat (depending on thickness) will keep your head warm. A jacket with a built-in hood is very good for long lift rides on cold, windy days. It's also extremely important to keep the back of your neck warm and flexible. A cold neck can tighten your back and shoulder muscles, contributing to overall tightness. When that happens, it becomes difficult to balance properly on the center of the skis.

- **Body.** A first layer of thin fleece or silk keeps moisture away from the skin and insulates the body. Choose shirts that are long enough to cover your lower back.

- **Hands.** Gloves and mittens come in many different designs and materials. Cow or goat hides with Thinsulate™ or Thermolite™ insulation are common in high-quality gloves. Cordura™ nylon gloves are also available and even come with waterproof membranes. Skiers who have difficulty staying warm should consider mittens, as there is nothing better for keeping the hands warm.

- **Legs.** Close fitting tights made from polypropylene make a good first layer; a looser-fitting second layer of fleece works well to keep you insulated from cold. On warm days, omit the second layer. An outer layer of waterproof, windproof material is an important last guard against the elements and an important piece of equipment.

- **Feet.** For best results in ski boots, wear thin- to medium-thickness ski-specific socks with micro fiber. They wick moisture and are knit tightly enough to hold heat. Thick socks made with wool are less effective because they compromise fit and comfort. Neoprene ski boots covers are making a comeback. They are easy to use and increase foot warmth by about 30 percent without batteries. Boot heaters are very popular and effective if you have difficulty keeping your feet warm. Proper boot fitting and carefully designed foot beds can also increase circulation and provide much better foot warmth. We've seen many skiers with chronically cold feet become very comfortable with proper foot beds.

Altitude

High altitude and dry air also affects skiers. Many Colorado and Western Mountain ski towns and ski areas are at well over 8,000 feet; the ski areas are usually higher. Spending even short periods of time at a high altitude can cause discomfort at best, but Acute Mountain Sickness (AMS) can also be a danger. AMS is caused by the body's intolerance of the atmospheric pressure and lower amounts of relative oxygen in the air at high altitudes. It can cause light-headedness, dizziness, nausea, headaches, and insomnia and usually occurs at altitudes above 7,000 feet. So it isn't unusual for someone coming from a lower lying area experience some degree of

AMS. The good news is that there are steps you can take to help yourself adjust to the higher altitudes of the mountains.

- **Stay away from alcohol,** at least until your body has had a chance to adjust to altitude and the additional stress of skiing all day. If you have no altitude symptoms it is probably alright to drink alcohol in moderation. In any case drink in moderation and supplement any alcoholic beverage with equal amounts of water.

- **Drink twice as much water as you do at home.** This will reduce the effects of dry air and dehydration due to exercise.

- **Eat foods that are light and easy to digest,** such as pasta, vegetables, fruits, and grains.

- **Try to take it easy the first day.** Maybe go shopping or take an easy stroll through the village.

- **Difficulty breathing, a feeling of having fluid in your lungs,** bluing of the lips, continued headaches, or dizziness are symptoms that mean you should get to lower altitude and see a doctor. Sometimes staying a night back at five thousand feet helps the body recover. If you have experienced altitude sickness in the past, choose lodgings at lower altitude and drive to the ski resorts.

Stretch 10 Minutes, Save $1300

Think stretching is a waste of precious time? Consider how much you've paid for your annual ski vacation:

5-day lift ticket	$250
4-day condo rental	$700
Airfare	$350
Total	**$1300**

Now imagine yourself pulling your hamstring on the first run of your first day and spending the rest of your vacation on the sofa in the condo. Taking 10 minutes to stretch doesn't seem like such a bad idea, does it?

Sunlight

At high altitudes, the effects of the sun are heightened by the thinness of the air. Overexposure to the sun's ultraviolet (UV) radiation can damage your skin and eyes. Effects of skin and eye damage include freckling, tanning, sun-burning,

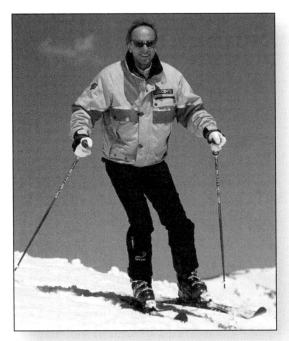

wrinkling, cataracts, and skin cancer. UV exposure is the most important environmental factor in the development of skin cancer. So before you step outside, remember the following.

• **Limit your time in the sun.** Take the greatest precautions between 10:00 A.M. and 4:00 P.M., the hours when UV rays are most intense.

• **Wear sunglasses or goggles** with 100 percent UV protection.

• **Chose a sunscreen with a Sun Protection Factor (SPF) of 15 or greater.** The higher the SPF, the longer the sunscreen's protection will last. Use sunscreen liberally and reapply it often; every two hours is recommended.

• **Choose water-resistant sunscreens** that won't wash off easily.

• **Use sunscreen with a current date.** Sunscreens have a shelf life of 2 to 3 years and some have an expiration date.

• **Apply sunscreen 30 minutes before going out in the sun** so that it has time to be absorbed into your skin.

Flexology: The Biomechanics of Skiing

The downhill skier is an example of forces at play: the internal forces of joints, muscles, ligaments, and tendons, contracting, elongating and stabilizing; and the external forces of wind, snow, friction, and gravity, which challenge the skier's skill and physical conditioning. A skier must stay focused on the work at hand in an ever-changing, complex, and sometimes chaotic environment. Preparing for all this takes a little more than just bending over at the waist and touching your toes three or four times and calling it a warm-up. A skier must have not only great endurance and physical and cardiovascular strength, but also a great deal of flexibility.

Flexspots

Moving your body down a mountain in a fluid, balanced, and efficient way involves a series of movements. Think of your body as a steel-link chain. A movement in any one part of the chain will continue through all the other parts until the energy is absorbed or dissipated. That's known as the "kinetic chain" and that's why Ski Flex focuses on overall flexibility and includes exercises for the upper body as well as for the legs and trunk.

Some areas of the body are particularly important to this overall flexibility. They're called "flexspots." Your flexspots are:

- **Neck.** During your runs, you are putting constant stress on your neck. Warm up by relaxing the neck and preparing it for stresses of pounding down the moguls.

- **Upper Back and Shoulders.** Increased flexibility here allows for greater range of motion of your arms, resulting in more fluid pole action and support for upper body stabilizing and balancing.

- **Upper Arms.** Focusing on this area will help you to keep your upper body properly focused for each turn and in a stable position to absorb surface irregularities. Keeping the arms in a proper home base position supports balance and timing for pole movement in each turn.

- **Lower Back and Trunk.** The lower back is your center of balance and provides strength and stability to your turns. When you bend, straighten, and control the upper body as you ski, you rely heavily on back stabilization and movement. The back muscles are in constant contraction while you are skiing. It is essential to keep them warm and flexible. This is definitely the most crucial area for a skier to keep flexible and healthy.

- **Inner Thigh (adductors) and Outer Hips (external rotators).** One of the most important things you do while skiing is transfer weight from one side of your body to the other. Stretching your hips is essential to preventing injury during the crucial weight transfers. These muscles are active for every turn as they help to tilt the skis on edge and release the skis from their edges. They must remain flexible and move independently from the lower back muscles. The adductors on the inner thigh help to engage the downhill ski and also adjust edging; therefore, tight adductors influence your overall ski security.

• **Hands and Wrists.** Prepare and warm up your hands and wrists for the impact they experience every time your poles touch the ground. Poles that are too long and too stiff may cause wrist problems. We recommend more flexible pole shafts for those skiers experiencing wrist problems.

• **Hamstrings and Quadriceps.** Your hamstrings and quadriceps act as shock absorbers on every bump and regulate pressure during every turn. Not only will tight hamstrings and quadriceps fatigue and tighten your legs, they will also affect your lower back and hips, considerably restricting your range of movement and your ability to transfer your weight in a fluid manner. It is also important to keep a full range of motion in your legs to release out of turns. Stiff quads and hamstrings damage your turn transition efficiency, affecting your skiing technique and reducing enjoyment.

• **Calves, Achilles Tendon, and Ankles.** Constantly controlling fore/aft balance and holding yourself upright in your ski boots can easily fatigue and cramp your calves. Stretching before and after you ski will help prepare your muscles for the task of omnidirectional movement and eliminate soreness.

The Mechanics of Skiing

Let's take a look at the mechanics of a ski turn and how improving your flexibility can create more fluidity, power, and control.

The transition of a turn is where most of the action occurs. This part of skiing requires the use of many joints in your body. The more joints available for use in a movement, the more consistent your natural movements become. And when your joints are moving fluidly you're able to line up your body to accept the forces of skiing. Remember that in skiing we use our muscles to align the skele-

The Anatomy of a Turn

Efficient and effective ski turns or skiing occurs when flexibility is available at the right time.
Proper timing develops a powerful stance and ski edge, giving us control and ease of turns.

Shoulders, upper back and arms keep the upper body in balance and generate the movements for pole plants.

The muscles of the lower back hold the upper body in place to maintain balance and help to create counteracting movements to resist rotary forces created in skiing.

The muscles on the outside and back of the hip or butt of the inside ski help to tilt the ski further on edge to compliment the outside ski.

Once in the turn, the quadriceps support the body and maintain stance.

The muscles higher up in the legs follow the tipping action and provide strength and power to the primary actions of the foot and ankle.

The hamstrings help to keep your feet under your body and are also the stabilizing muscles used for absorbing bumps.

Your knees and legs follow the actions of the skis and boots.

The muscles on the inside of the thigh of the downhill leg help tip the skis more aggressively once the turn has begun.

You begin a ski turn using muscles attached to the foot and ankle to tip or tilt the boots and skis to angle them to the surface.

ton. When the skeleton is properly stacked or aligned for each turn the body can easily absorb forces and we therefore ski with less fatigue. If we are late in moving and slow to react because of stiff or non-functioning muscles, we overuse other muscles. Muscle overuse leads to fatigue and the possibility of injury. Efficient and effective ski turns or skiing occurs when flexibility is available at the right time. Proper timing develops a powerful stance and ski edge, giving us control and ease of turns. (See photograph, page 15.)

- You begin a ski turn using muscles in the foot and ankle to tip or tilt the boots and skis to angle them to the surface.

- Your knees and legs follow the actions of the skis and boots.

- The muscles higher up in the legs follow the tipping action and provide strength and power to the primary actions of the foot and ankle.

- The muscles on the inside of the thigh of the downhill leg help tip the skis more aggressively once the turn has begun.

- The muscles on the outside and back of the hip or butt of the inside ski help to tilt the ski further on edge to compliment the outside ski.

- Once in the turn, the quadriceps support the body and maintain stance.

- The hamstrings help to keep your feet under your body and are also the stabilizing muscles used for absorbing bumps.

- The muscles of the lower back hold the upper body in place to maintain balance and help to create counteracting movements to resist rotary forces created in skiing.

- Shoulders, upper back and arms keep the upper body in proper balance and generate the movements for pole plants.

Once a turn nears completion the legs flex to absorb the turn and tilt the skis in the new direction to begin the next turn. Again, all the muscles that tilted the skis for the first turn must now reverse their action, release the tilting. and return to neutral position between turns. This requires strong flexing, or bending of the legs, using the quadriceps muscles group.

SKI FLEX

While in transition between turns the lower back keeps the upper body stable and the arms and shoulders are used for pole plant movements and stabilizing of the rotary forces.

You can see that the whole body is involved in skiing and that all the joints and muscles need to act in conjunction. A stiff muscle group can throw the whole program out of whack. A complete warm-up and stretch before putting on ski gear and after ski gear is in place are part of the Ski Flex program. World-class athletes warm up everyday before skiing. Why shouldn't we recreational and amateur skiers do the same?

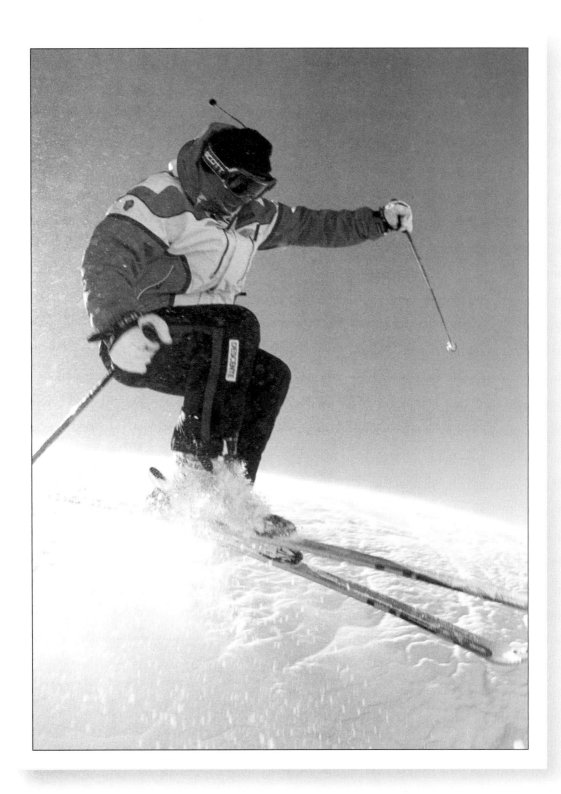

Part 2: The Ski Flex Program

SOME SKIERS DO A COUPLE OF WARM-UPS AND STRETCHES BEFORE THEY race out the door to ski. But once they're outside, they neglect to continue warming up. Other skiers wait until they're on the slopes with their boots on to do any warming up. They march up and down for a bit or do some torso twists and consider it done. Neither approach is complete. Warming up and stretching is a process that should start indoors, continue on once you're outdoors—and even through your first run of the day. That's why Ski Flex program is comprised of four components:

1. Indoor Warm-Ups and Stretches;
2. Stretches you do On the Snow with Skis Off;
3. Exercises you do On the Snow with Skis On; and
4. Stretches you during your First Runs of the Day.

The result? A total body flexibility workout.

It's a good idea to read through all the following exercises before beginning and to follow some advice: Stretching is not a competition. What you don't achieve today may come tomorrow. But it takes commitment. Stay on the path. Oftentimes, people who are naturally talented in some activity never achieve greatness because they quit at the first obstacle, so don't give up.

And now, to Ski Flex!

Indoor Warm-Ups and Stretches

Before stretching, it's important to warm up to get the blood flowing into the muscles you are about to stretch. Many individuals jog or walk as a warm-up. Although both these activities will increase the core temperature, the movements of jogging and walking are not similar to the complex movement demanded by downhill skiing. Downhill skiers move their bodies in all ranges of motion: side to side (frontal), rotational (transverse), and front and back (saggetal). Doesn't it make more sense to warm up using the same movements required in skiing? These pre-ski indoor warm-ups target the specific muscles (quadriceps, hamstrings, gluteus, calves, torso, shoulders) and movements required for skiing and prepare them for the task at hand—skiing—not jogging or walking.

Standing Warm-Ups

These two exercises begin to get your hip and knee joints warmed up and ease your whole body into movement. If you feel very tight—as you may if you've just rolled out of bed—be sure to take things slowly and gently.

The Exercises

Knee *and* **Hip Circles**

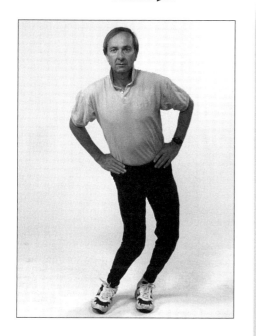 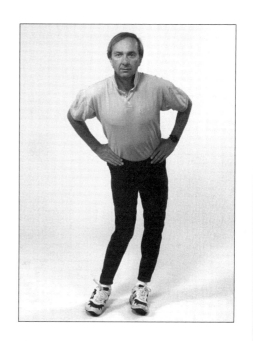

Warms up: Legs, ankles, lower back

Reps: 20 rotations in each direction

This continual-movement warm-up involves flexing or bending both knees and moving them in a circle. Try making a circle around your feet with your knee leading the movements. Your legs must come almost straight as they move back under the hips. When the knees are at the front of the circle they are the most bent. The front of the circle is directly forward when you are looking straight ahead. Imagine a circle drawn on the floor around your feet and make your knees go around to follow the line of the circle. Once you begin to really flex the knees and roll the legs, you will feel your shoes coming up on their edges like you would with your skis.

Upper Body Circles

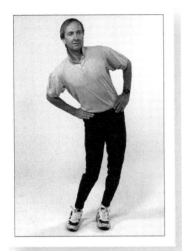
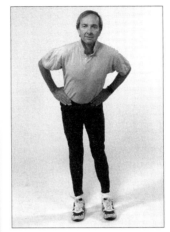
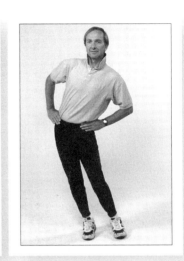

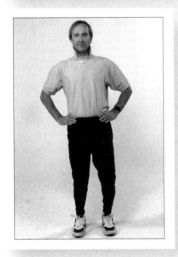

Warms up: Lower back, hips; stretches hamstrings

Reps: 20 rotations in each direction

Upper body rotations are the same circular actions as the Knee and Hip Circles on the previous page but with the legs kept straight and the upper body rotated at the hip. This movement is like a Hula-Hoop swinging of the hips. If you can stick your butt out to the back and each side as far as you can while making circles, you are on the right track.

Floor Warm-Ups

Flexibility and warming up go together; when the muscles are warm they are more likely to stretch without pain or resistance. The lower back can stiffen up easily when skiing. All the bumps and twisting movements in skiing added to the cold and sitting on the chairlift surely contribute to a stiff back. Begin each of these exercises—which target your back, abs, torso, and legs—slowly and work up to your best range of motion. Try to remember and keep track of your range of motion at the beginning and end of the exercises. Also keep track of your progress over a period of weeks or during skiing weekends or vacation. Keep in mind that it's common for your range of motion to decrease after a few days of skiing because of muscle tension. It is important to do these exercises even when you are not skiing. Your muscles will be much more likely to respond to stretching if they're accustomed to proper warm-up exercises.

The Exercises

Toe Touches

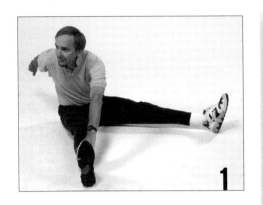

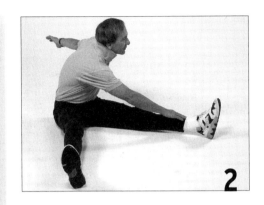

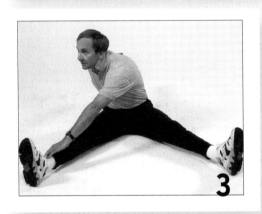

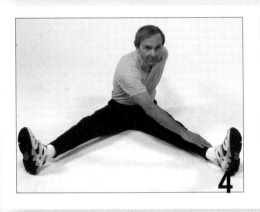

Warms up: Back, hamstrings   **Reps:** 20 to 30 each side

This is a warm-up and stretching exercise. Slowly reach forward until your hands are over your ankles. Reach your right hand over to your left foot while moving your left hand and arm behind your back, keeping the arms straight. Now reverse the movement, bringing your left hand forward and reaching toward the right ankle or foot (depending on your flexibility, you may not touch your foot). Continue alternating touches. Once your breathing quickens, stop and hold each toe reach for five seconds. Each time you should feel your lower back stretch and the muscles behind your legs and close to the floor giving way and allowing for greater range of motion and stretch. This stretch should never be forced. Keep your lower back covered and warm during the whole exercise. Note: Remember that depending on your natural flexibility, you may never actually touch your toes.

The Swimmer

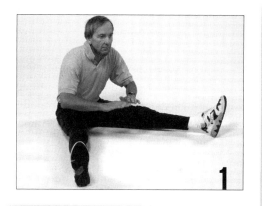

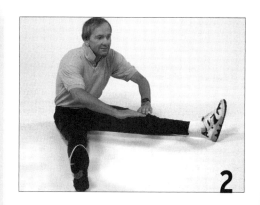

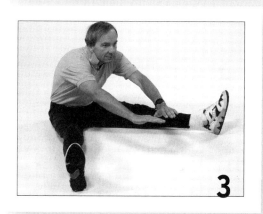

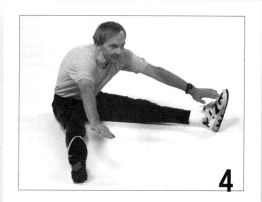

Warms up: Lower back, hamstrings, glutes

Reps: 5 to 10

This stretch is similar to the breaststroke in swimming. Begin slowly and don't try to reach too far at first. Stay within your comfort zone, which means not reaching to the point of pain. Pain should not be part of these exercises; it only causes your muscles and tendons to react by tightening.

Beginner Torso Twist

Warms up (and strengthens):
Lower back, abs

Reps: 8 to 12

Lie on the floor with knees flexed and thighs perpendicular to the floor. Spread your arms to the side for stability and to keep your lower back on the floor. You may have to push your arms against the floor to keep the upper body from moving. Move your legs to one side until one knee touches the floor on one side (do not keep your knees together), and then bring legs back starting position. Move your legs to the other side and touch the other knee to the floor. the other leg and knee to the floor. Now alternate until you achieve eight to 12 touches on each side.

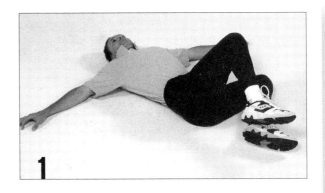

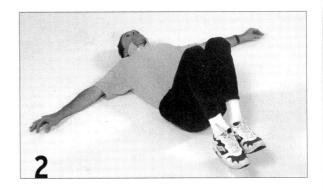

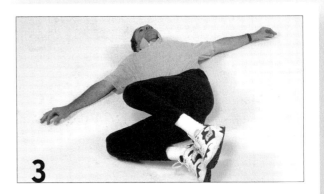

Advanced Torso Twist

Warms up (and strengthens):
Lower back, abs

Reps: 8 to 12

Lie on the floor with knees flexed and thighs perpendicular to the floor. Spread your arms to the side for stability and to keep your lower back on the floor. You may have to push your arms against the floor to keep the upper body from moving. Keeping your knees together, touch both legs to one side and then bring them back up and then touch them to the other side. This exercise is both a warm up and lower back and abdominal stretcher and strengthener.

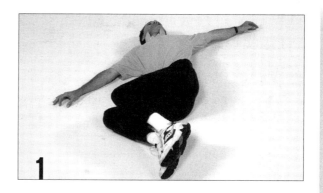

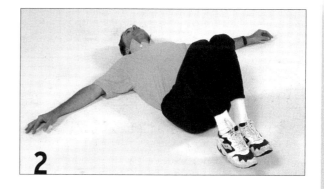

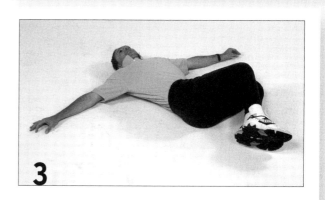

Leg Lifts

Warms up (and strengthens):
Upper quads and hip flexor

Reps: 8 to 10

From a seated position with your hands and arms behind your hips for support, extend your legs, while keeping them off the floor. Bring the legs back to the flexed starting position. Repeat this movement at least eight to 10 times. This is a warm-up as well as a muscle strengthener.

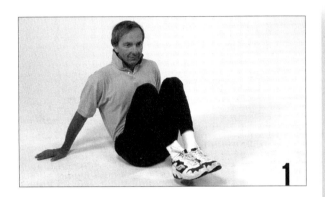

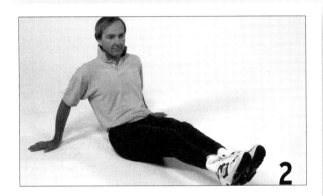

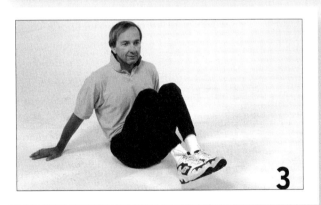

Leg Crossovers

Warms up (and stretches):
Glutes, lower back

Reps: 5 to 7 in each direction

From a seated position raise one leg
and swing it over the other leg.
Keeping the leg straight, point the toe
up toward the shoulders and away
from the body. Roll up on the opposite
hip and hold. Now swing the leg back
to the starting position and lift and
swing the other leg over and out to
the side. Repeat in both directions
five to seven times in each direction.

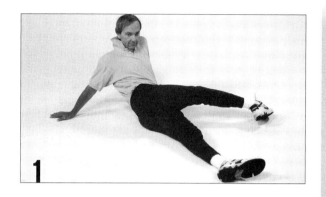

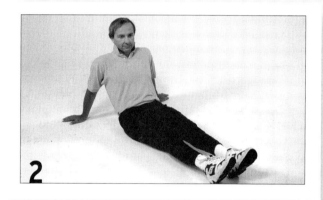

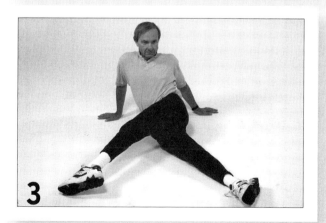

Crossover Quad Stretch

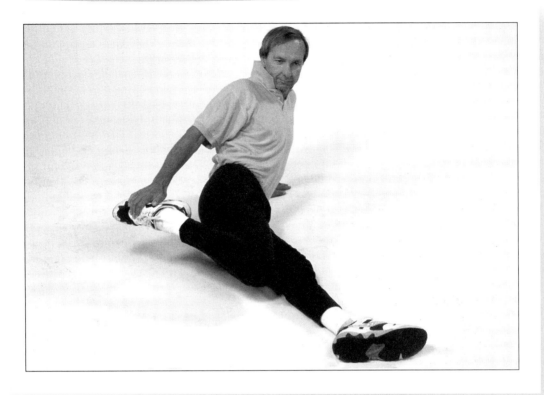

Warms up (and stretches): Quads

Reps: 5 each side

After finishing the Leg Crossovers (page 30), it's convenient (and effective) to stretch your quad muscles from the same position. While seated, roll over onto one hip and hold the ankle of the top leg. Bend the leg and then gradually and gently pull the ankle up and back to your butt. Feel the gradual stretch of the quad muscles as you hold that position, keeping some pressure on the ankle to keep the knee flexed.

Stretches

By now you should be all warmed up. (If you're still a little tight, ride a stationary bike or use a Stairmaster.) Once you begin the following stretches, make sure you stay warm by moving fluidly from one stretch into another, never resting for too long in one position. These stretches will elevate your core temperature, help you stretch dynamically in a full range of motion, and charge up your neuromuscular system.

The following exercises focus on two types of stretching: static and dynamic. Static stretching requires simply holding a stretch for 10 to 20 seconds. The next set of exercises start with static stretching, which helps you get used to each stretch and recognize which muscles are involved.

With that accomplished, you can move on to dynamic stretching, which involves actively moving into a stretch, holding it for three to five seconds, and then repeating the motion five times. With each motion, the stretch gets deeper and deeper. This doesn't mean "bouncing" or "jerking" into a stretch; it means simulating the kind of motions you will most likely make as you move down the slope. Such stretches incorporate twisting your torso, for example.

The best pre-ski stretching is dynamic stretching, because it also serves as a warm-up. Once you've performed each of the following stretches

The 9 Cardinal Rules of Stretching

Keep these simple points in mind anytime you stretch.
1. Breathe. Never hold your breath.
2. Stand up straight. Maintain good posture.
3. Move gently. Never bounce or jerk.
4. Never force or strain your muscles when you stretch.
5. Maintain consistency.
6. Stay in touch with your body and focus on the muscles being stretched.
7. Never over-stretch (i.e., pushing into a painful stretch).
8. Consult a doctor before beginning any flexibility program.
9. Smile and relax.

statically and feel comfortable doing them, perform them dynamically before you hit the slopes. Repeat each stretch several times, and then try to move quickly from one stretch into the next. This will get your heart pumping and your muscles warmed up, and it will make the stretching program go quickly so you can take off down the mountain. Throughout the exercises, keep in mind *The 9 Cardinal Rules of Stretching* (page 31).

The Exercises

Yes *and* No

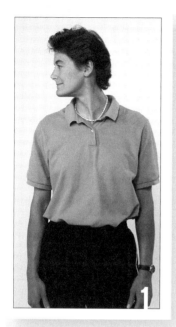 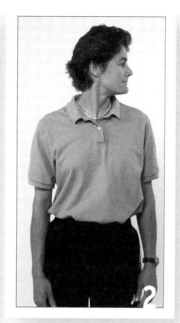 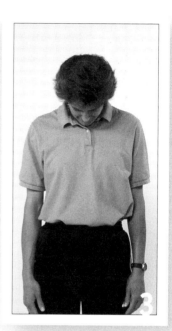

Stretches: Neck   **Reps:** 5

Start with your head in a neutral, face-forward position. Nod your head "Yes" by bringing your chin to your chest, then return it back to the neutral position. Be careful not to extend the neck backward! Turn your head "No" gently to each side as shown, until your chin is over your shoulder. Repeat this stretch five times.

Neck Rotations

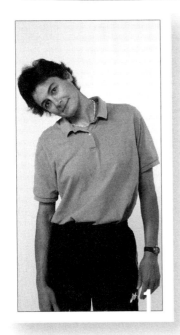 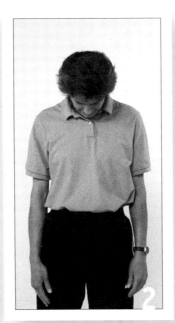 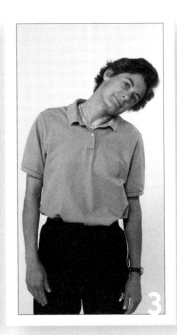

Stretches: Neck   **Reps:** 5

Start with your head in a neutral, face-forward position. Slowly and gently tilt your head toward your right shoulder and then rotate it in a counter-clockwise manner to the left shoulder and then repeat in the opposite direction.

Forearm Flex *and* Stretch

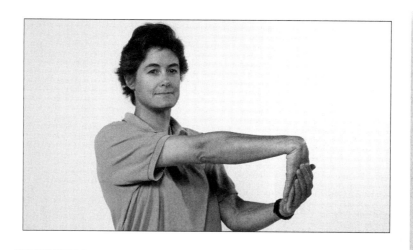

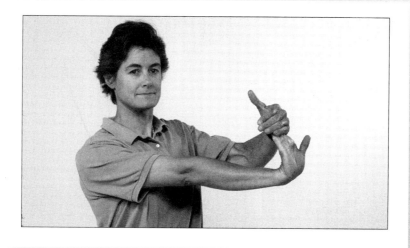

Stretches: Forearm   **Reps:** 5 on each hand

With one arm extended in front of you, gently pull your fingers back with your palm facing outward. Reverse the motion by pressing your fingers down with your opposite hand, palms inward. The forearm flex and stretch helps your skiing by preparing your forearms for the impact of your poles on the snow.

Quads Knee Flex

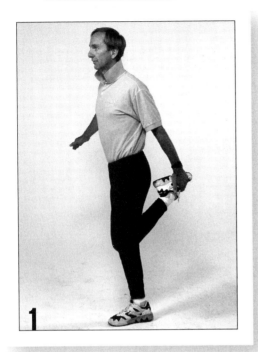 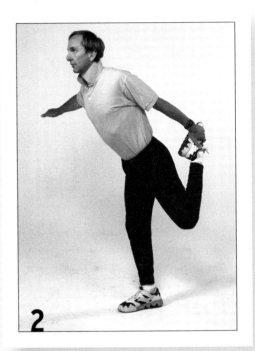

Stretches: Quadriceps

Reps: 3 to 5 on each leg

Balance on one leg. Grab the foot or ankle of the opposite leg with your hand. Gently pull your leg back and under your hips. Hold for a few seconds (fig. 1). You can also stretch the hip flexors by extending the hip and raising the heel of the foot behind your hips (fig. 3). Alternate legs and perform three to five times on each leg. It can be difficult to hold your balance when first learning this stretch. Use the wall or a friend until you can perform the exercise by yourself.

Hamstring Stretcher

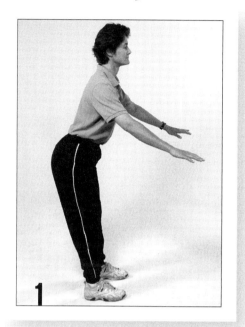

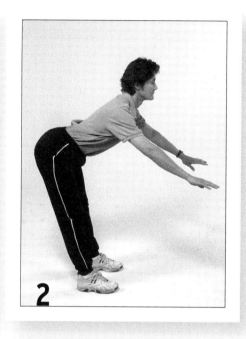

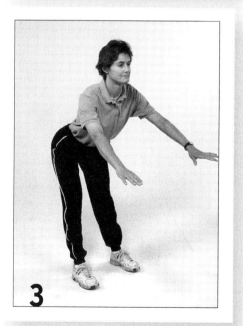

Stretches: Hamstrings

Reps: 2

Bend forward at the waist, keeping your stomach tight and your back flat. Do not bounce. Bend until you can feel the stretch and then hold for 10 seconds. Repeat twice. Tight hamstrings can mean a tight back, too, which adversely affects the fluidity of your turns.

Side Lunges

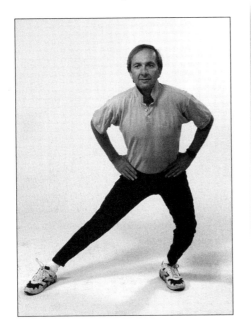 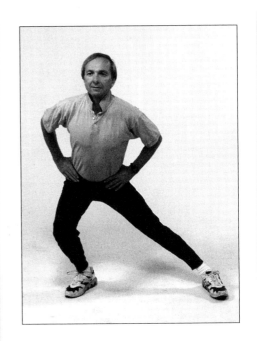

Stretches: Inner thigh (adductors)

Reps: 4

Stand with your feet more than shoulder width apart; rest your hands on your hips for support. Keep one leg straight and then bend the other leg. Hold for 10 seconds. Switch legs and repeat four times. For a more challenging stretch, place your hands on the floor between your legs.

Rooster Crow

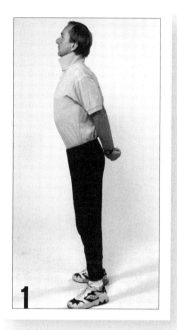 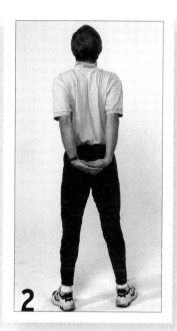 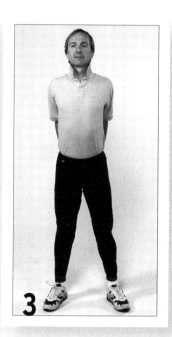

Stretches: Chest, shoulders, upper arms

Reps: 2 to 3

Interlace your fingers behind your back with palms facing up. Squeeze your shoulder blades together as you stick out your chest and press your hands backward. Look toward the ceiling, contract your butt, and stretch the front of your shoulders and chest. A slight arch in your back will increase this stretch. When stretching, remember that your ears and shoulders are mortal enemies. Keep your shoulders down. Combine with the Tree-Hugger stretch and repeat two or three times.

Tree Hugger

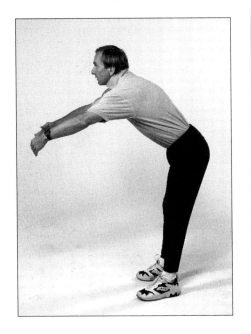 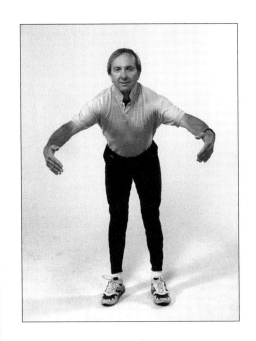

Stretches: Upper and lower back

Reps: 5

With your feet about shoulder width apart, pretend you're wrapping your arms around a big tree. Keep your chin off of your chest as you contract your stomach muscles. Be sure to keep your abdominal muscles tight. You will feel this stretch from your tailbone to the top of your head.

Back *and* Side Stretchers

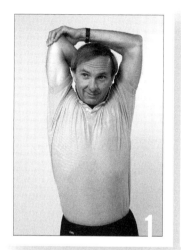

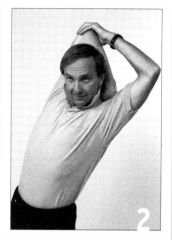

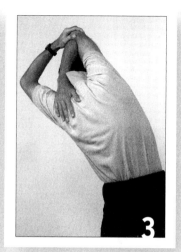

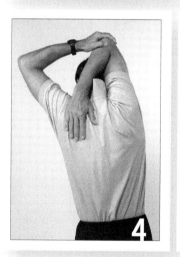

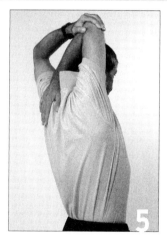

Stretches:
Back and sides

Reps: 8 on each side

Reach one elbow up toward the ceiling and your hand behind your neck and toward the opposite shoulder. With the other hand, assist the stretch by gently pulling back on the elbow. Bend at the waist to stretch your side. Repeat eight times on each side.

Calf *and* Shin Stretches

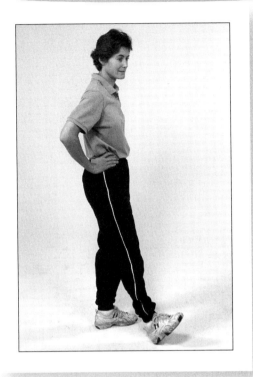 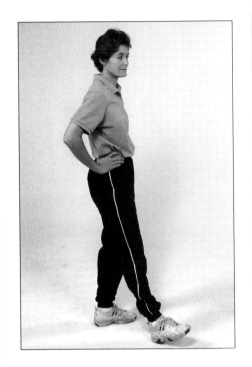

Stretches: Calf and shin

Reps: 3 on each leg

The calf and anterior tibialis opposing muscles are located in the lower leg on the front and back of the shin below the knee. They're important in skiing because they offer control and allow balance in a fore/aft range. Simply placing the leg out front with your shoe on its heel will put you in the starting position. As you pull your toe toward your shin you stretch the calf and contract the tibialis anterior. Extending the toe toward the floor will stretch the tibialis and contract the calf. Hold each position for approximately five seconds.

Cobra

Stretches: Abs, lower back, arms

Reps: 2

The cobra is done with assistance from the arms; it's essential that you don't force the arms into the extension. Begin by lying on your chest. Place your forearms flat on the floor while raising your shoulders. This is your beginning position. Slowly extend your arms as you arch your back. Do not push your back if you feel resistance or if your back becomes stiff and movement is restricted. Hold this position and then slowly lower yourself back to the ground, repeating the movements.

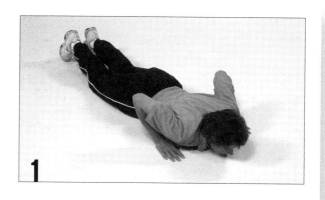

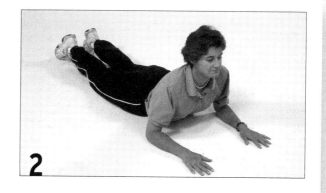

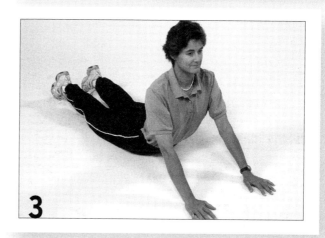

Ankle Stretch

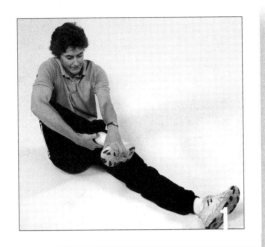

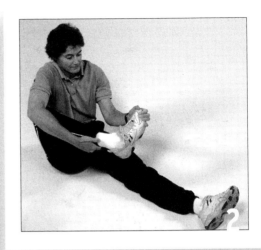

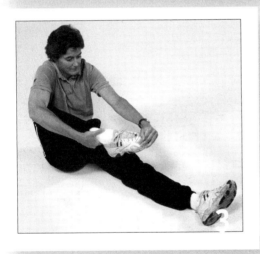

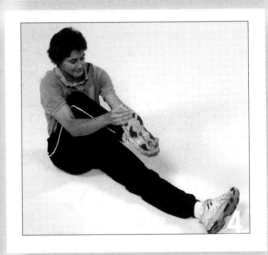

Stretches: Ankle   **Reps:** 2

The muscles that control lower leg tipping action are on the outside of the lower leg and the back of the leg. The tendons for these muscles run along the outside of the ankle and attach under the foot. They're difficult to stretch and have limited range of motion. One way to access the range of motion of these muscles is to manually rotate the ankle in circles, slowly creating flexibility. Grab your toes and slowly rotate the foot in a circle. Bring the toes toward your shin as far as you can and also press the toes down away from the shin at the bottom of the circle. Hold the leg with the other hand as you work the ankle to full range in every direction.

Hip Socket Stretch

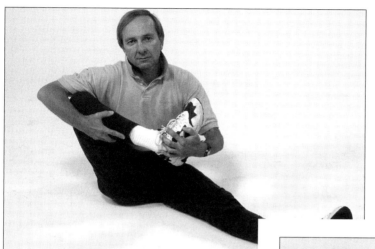

Stretches: Hip

Reps: 1 on each leg

From a seated position, extend your right leg fully forward. Bend your left leg, grasping the heel with your right hand and cradling your left leg with your left arm. Apply gentle, even pressure to your left leg as you pull it towards you. Relax your breath and be careful not to overstretch.

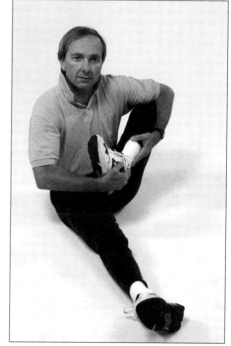

Corkscrew

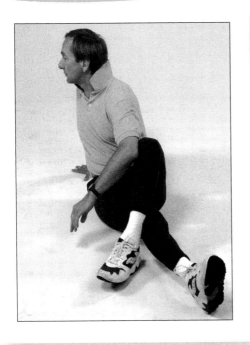 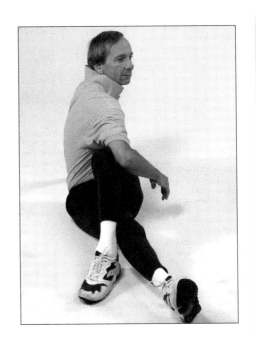

Stretches: Glutes, lower back

Reps: 2 on each side

Sit with your right leg straight. Cross your left foot over your right leg and place your left foot flat on the floor by your right knee. Keep your back straight and don't slouch! Place your right hand behind you and your left arm inside your left knee. Turn and look toward your right hand. Without changing foot placement, switch hands and face the opposite direction. Hold each of these positions for 30 seconds. Switch legs and repeat.

Optional Add-Ons:
The Wall Sits

If you have the time or the inclination before you race out the door, you may want to include one or more of the following Wall Sit exercises in your routine. Wall Sits warm up your quadriceps and stretch the hip flexor muscles and glutes. You can also do them with your ski poles to simulate skiing positions. *Note:* It is important to keep your lower back and shoulders in contact with the wall while doing these stretches.

The Exercises

Wall Sit I

Stretches (and strengthens):
Quadriceps

Reps: 5

Stand with your heels approximately 18 inches from the wall. Keep your legs almost straight, and then flex or bend your legs, letting your back slide down the wall. When you have lowered your hips almost to a sitting position, begin pushing back up to the starting position. If you have a hard time pushing yourself back up, don't lower so far on the second rep. This is a great warm-up for the legs and also can be used to prepare for the ski season.

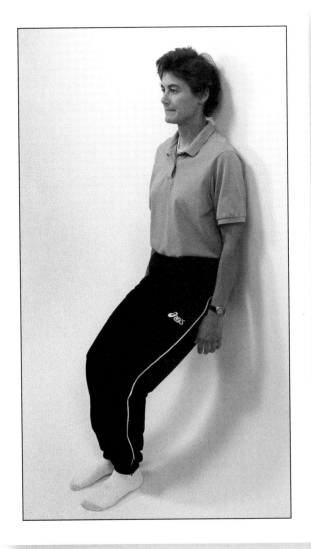

Wall Sit II

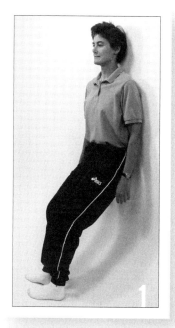 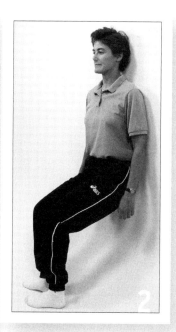 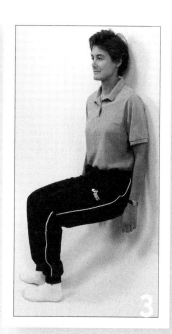

Stretches: Hip flexor, lower back, and glutes

Reps: 5

Stand with your heels approximately 18 inches from the wall. Keeping your entire back (including your hips) pressed tightly against the wall, turn both your feet as far as you can in one direction. Now allow your back to slide down the wall as you flex your legs and then push yourself back up. Turn your feet in the other direction and repeat.

Wall Sit III

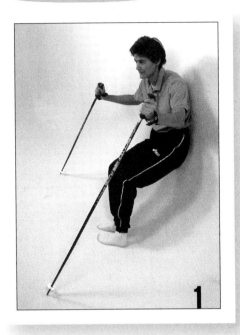

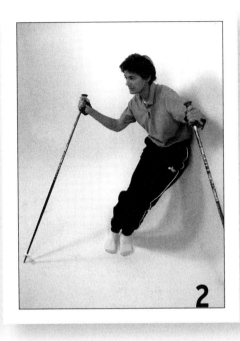

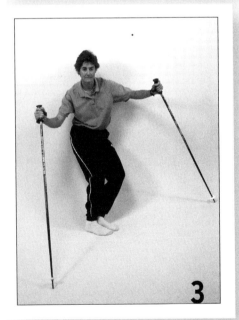

Stretches: Hip flexor, lower back, and glutes

Reps: 2 to 3

Grab your ski poles for this one. Wall Sit III is great for experiencing the flexibility and position needed to keep your body from rotating during a ski turn. This stretch can be used as a body orienting practice exercise for skiing movements. As in the other Wall Sit exercises you can flex and extend the legs to enhance and simulate actual leg movements during skiing.

On Snow with Skis Off

Ideally, stretching and warming up in ski boots should be done after you reach the top of your first lift ride. Find a flat spot away from the lift. Take off your skis and begin the warm-up exercises described here. We know you're eager, but remember: You're helping yourself to ski better, ski faster, and with less chance of injury.

The Exercises

Boot swing, page 52

Boot Circles, page 54

Arm Circles, page 56

Arm Swings, page 58

Lateral Lunges, page 59

Advanced Lunges, page 60

Lateral Tipping, page 61

The Curse of the Ski Boot

Try to avoid standing around in ski boots or walking in them for extended periods before skiing. Ski boots place your knees in a flexed position and limit your range of motion. You can become stiff and your muscles can tighten while you are standing around. During my years of ski coaching I noticed my lower back becoming stiff and painful. I first thought it was from lifting and setting gates for the racers, but I later discovered it was really due to all the standing on the slopes watching and coaching while in ski boots. Many coaches today use a soft mountaineering boot for the coaching and standing to protect their bodies.

Boot Swing

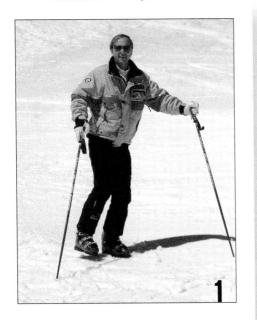

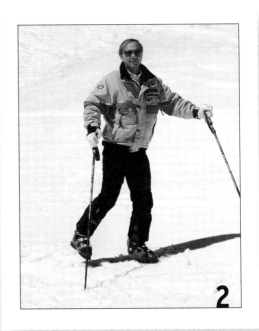

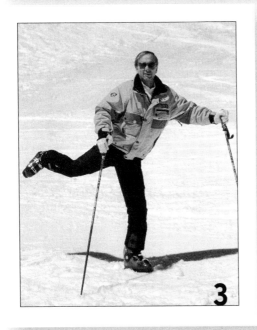

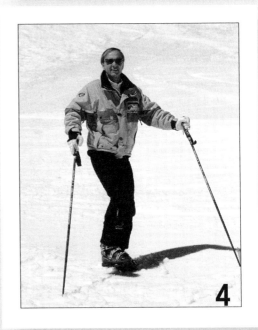

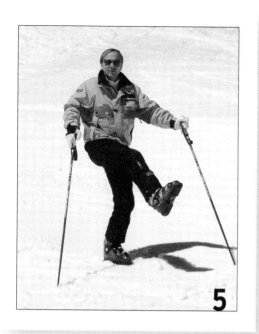
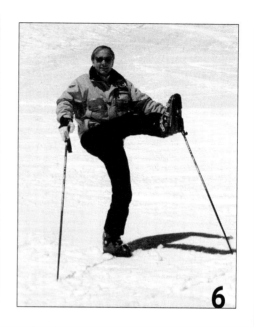

Stretches/Warms Up: Hips, glutes

Reps: 10 to 15 on each leg

Lean slightly to one side, using your poles to help you balance. Lift one leg straight behind your body, swing it forward as high as you can, and then swing it back. This is a very satisfying movement because you can feel the hip and glute muscles stretching and lengthening with the help of the weight of the boot.

Boot Circles

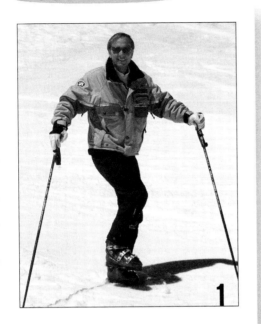

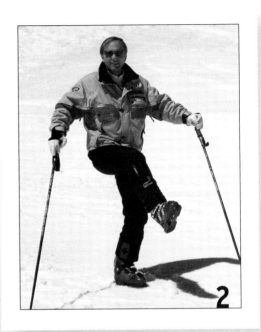

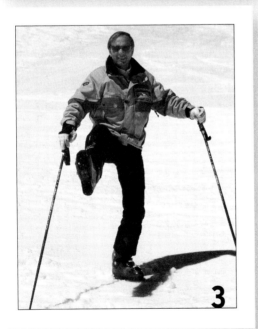

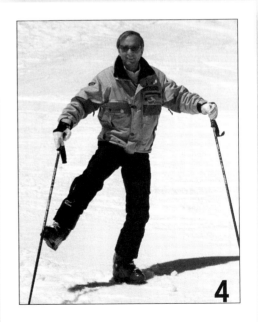

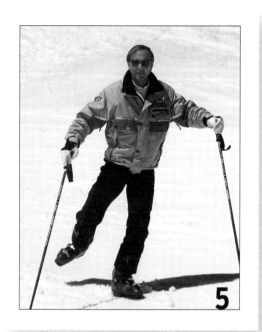

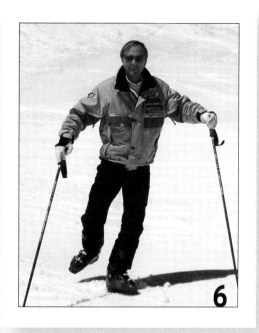

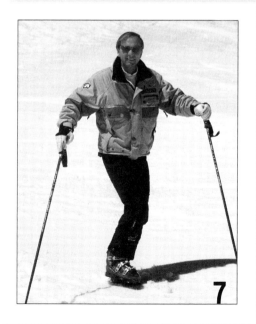

Stretches/Warms Up: Hips

Reps: 5 in each direction on each leg

Boot circles stretch and warm up the important muscles around the hip at both the front and back of the body. Start in the same stance as in the Boot Swings (page 52–53). Make a circle to the side of the body, lifting the boot as high to the side as you can. Do five circles in each direction with each leg. Continue these boot exercises diligently throughout the season and you'll find that you're strengthening the same muscles you're warming up and stretching.

Arm Circles

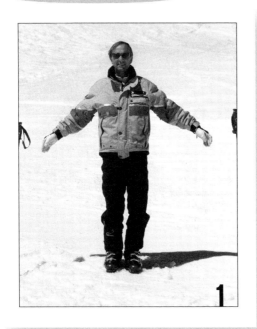

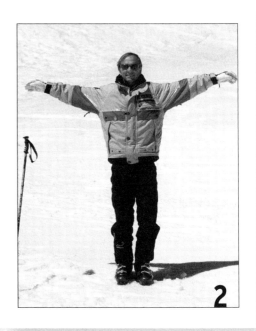

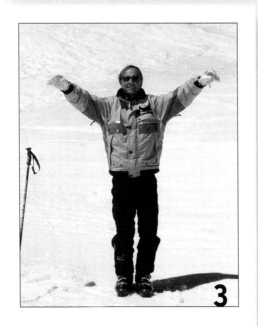

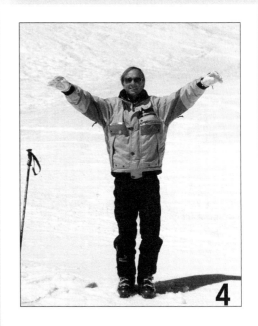

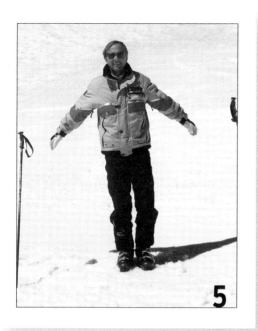

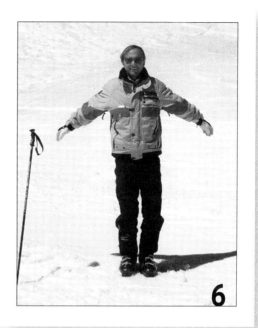

Stretches/Warms Up: Hips, glutes

Reps: 10 to 15 in each direction

Just like the Arm Swings on the next page, Arm Circles help your body react to changes in balance. Raise your arms to shoulder height and make large circles with both arms at the same time. Flex your legs as your arms come to the bottom of the circle; extend your legs as your arms come to the top. You can bounce slightly as you lift and drop your arms.

Arm Swings

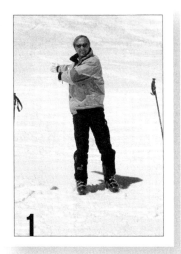
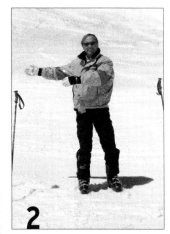
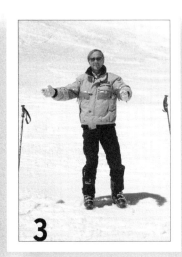
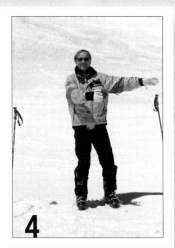
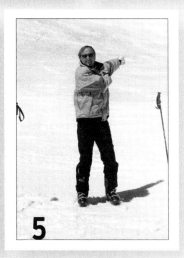

Stretches/Warms Up: Torso   **Reps:** 10 to 15 in each direction

Arm swings are important because they prepare you to deal with forces you'll have to resist and balance against as you ski. Stand with your boots about 12 inches apart and raise your arms to shoulder height. Swing both arms to one side as far as you can, following with your upper trunk, and then swing in the opposite direction. Do this with energy and conviction! You'll notice that you'll need to grip and maintain balance with your legs. Arm Swings help you prepare for the balance challenges to which you'll have to respond during the day on the slopes.

Lateral Lunges

Stretches/Warms Up:
Adductors, lower back, hips, quadriceps

Reps: 10 on each leg

This may be the most important leg warm-up you'll do before putting on your skis. Lateral Lunges give you flexibility and stretch the adductors, lower back, and hips. They also provide an important quadriceps warm-up. Since these movements are in the limited range of flexion that the ski boot provides, you'll need to use more hip, lower back, and knee flexion. Begin by standing with the boots three feet apart. Point your boots outward slightly. Flex, or bend, one leg and stretch the other to one side with your hands on your thighs. Hold most of your weight on the flexed leg. Once you reach a strongly flexed position, push yourself back to a standing position and then move right into the lunge on the other leg. Move from one side to the other at least 10 times.

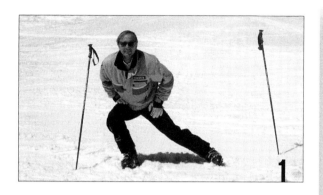

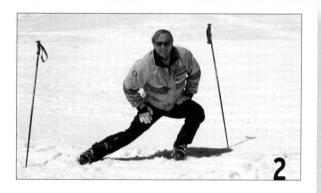

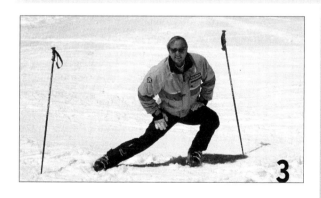

Advanced Lunges

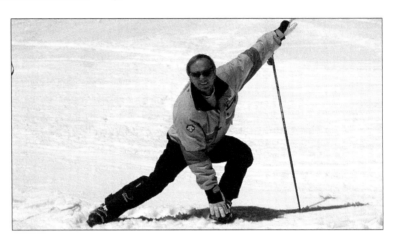

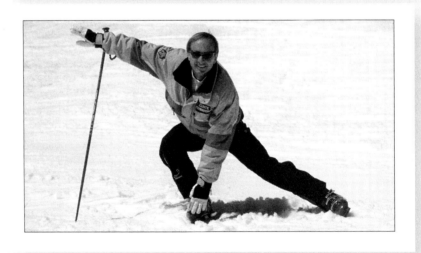

Stretches/Warms Up: Adductors, lower back, hips, quadriceps

Reps: 10 on each leg

In Advanced Lunges, you achieve additional benefit by reaching the hand opposite the flexed leg toward the boot of the flexed leg. Alternate touches, keeping your rhythm going for at least five reps in each direction. These will really warm you up on a cold day. (In fact if you feel cold *during* the day, pull over to a flat area and do this exercise; you'll feel better immediately!)

Lateral Tipping

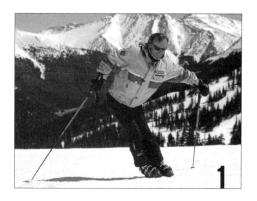

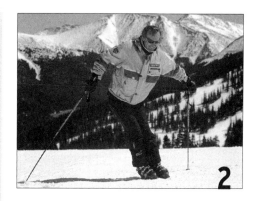

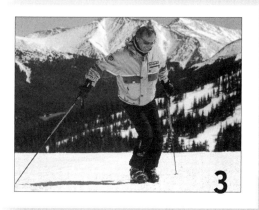

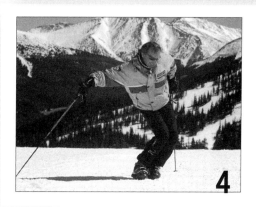

Stretches/Warms Up: Ankles   **Reps:** 10 on each leg

Innovations in ski design have changed skiing. Shaped skis make it easier to turn and provide higher performance, making skiing more enjoyable than at any other time in the sport's history. And because skiers can tip shaped skis more aggressively, they experience greater lateral loads on their body. We therefore include this lateral movement warm-up to prepare you for the required movements of shaped ski skiing. Stand with your boots together, using your poles for balance, if necessary. Tip both boots to one side; increase the angle by trying to place the boots on their sides. Your legs will follow the action you're performing with the boots. Move and practice this exercise in both directions, tipping your boots as far as you can. As a final move tip the boots quickly from one side to the other without stopping. Tip the boots 10 times without stopping to gain the best results from this warm-up.

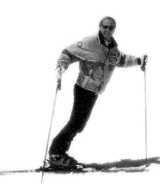

On Snow with Skis On

Once you've finished the last set of stretches, go ahead and put on your skis. These next stretches will help your balance, warm up your ankles, and even help you fit your boots.

The Exercises

Lateral Edging

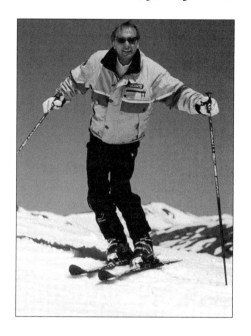 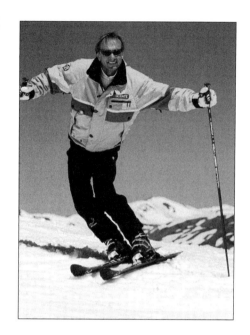

Benefits: Increases awareness of edging; prepares body to move with skis

Reps: 5 in each direction

This exercise is similar to Lateral Tipping (page 61), but it's done with skis on. Stand on the side of a slope that has a very slight incline. Use your poles for balance, if necessary. Tip your skis up onto the outside edge; continue to tip the skis until they're almost on their side walls. Hold this position for only a second, and then move back to a normal stance. Repeat at least five times on each side.

Shuffling

Benefits: Helps assess boot fit

Reps: 2 in each direction

Boots can get stiff in cold weather and, depending on how you buckle them, they may restrict your ankle range of motion. Shuffling lets you test your range before you ski. Stand on a flat area with boots and skis parallel. Move one boot forward and the other backward, sending the boots in opposite directions as far as they can move. Now reverse the action. Feel how much pressure is placed against the back of your calves and the front of your shins as you shuffle. If this is the same amount of pressure you feel when skiing, you're either too far back or forward on the boots. There are times when we need to be this far forward or back in the boots (such as when we're recovering from a balance miscue), but if you're leaning on your boots to the extent demonstrated by the extreme positions of this exercise, you're skiing out of balance. If you can't achieve enough ankle flexion, loosen your boot's top buckle. Many skiers overtighten that buckle and therefore restrict their ability to achieve proper forward pressure on the skis. Most modern boots have power straps that wrap around the top of the boot. These straps are provided to give better fit around the top of the ankle. One instant fix for an overly stiff boot is to wrap the power strap around the leg inside the plastic flap of the boot shell. Do up the power strap before you do up your buckles. After you have your power strap in place do up your buckles. The two middle buckles are the most important; they should be snug. The top buckle need not be as snug.

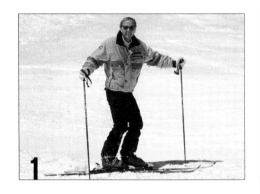

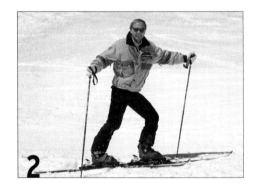

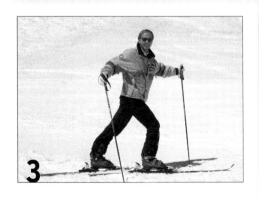

Fore/Aft Boot Test

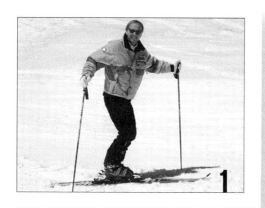
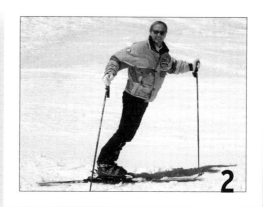
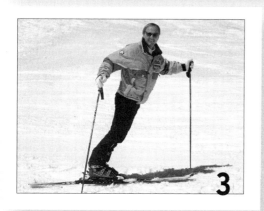
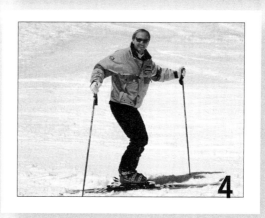

Benefits: Helps assess boot fit   **Reps:** 2 in each direction

The Fore/Aft boot test provides the same information as the Shuffle but in a different way. On a flat area, place your boots together, lean forward, and push your skis back under and behind your hips. Try to push and pull with your legs so the skis actually move on the snow. This is the same feeling you should have when recentering your body over your skis while skiing. Skiers rarely try to reposition to a forward or centered position before each turn. Experts are always adjusting balance while they ski. Build this recentering movement into every turn. Next, test the backward range by pushing your feet forward until you sense that you're leaning and being supported by the back of the boots. This is a position—often called the "back seat"—is a position you don't want to be skiing in. (For more detailed fore/aft skiing movements, see *Anyone Can Be an Expert Skier 2*, by Harald Harb.

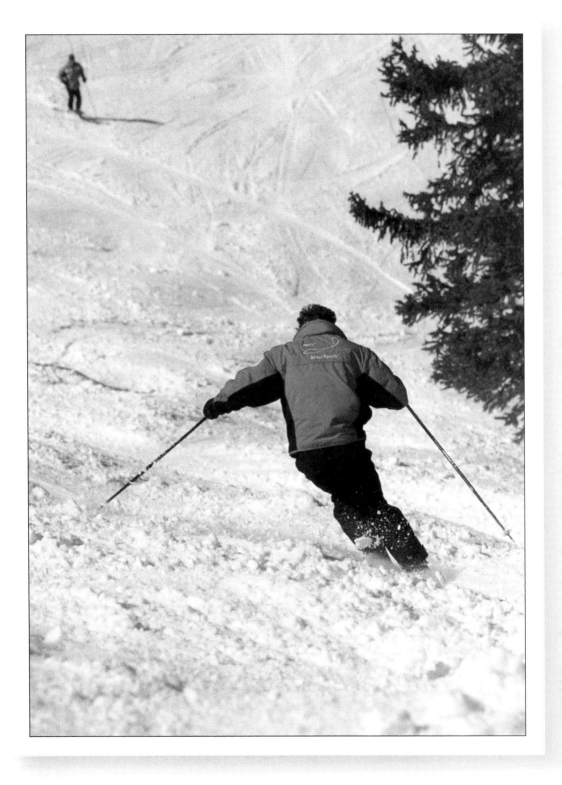

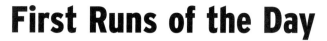

First Runs of the Day

It's important to be completely warmed up and aware of your balance before you attack the slopes. You can avoid many injuries by being properly prepared. Most of the exercises presented here can give you important feedback about how you stand on your skis. A centered, properly balanced stance can help you avoid many common, minor injuries and even help you to avoid more severe knee injuries. Rarely have skiers been injured while skiing in control and balanced. Use these exercises to develop a better sense of balance on your skis.

The Exercises

Balancing

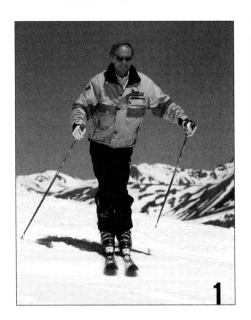

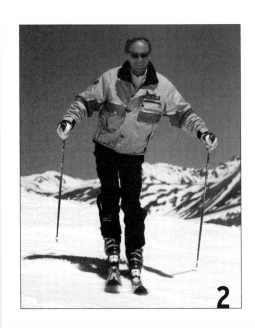

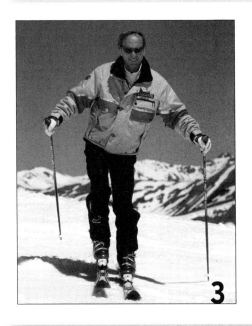

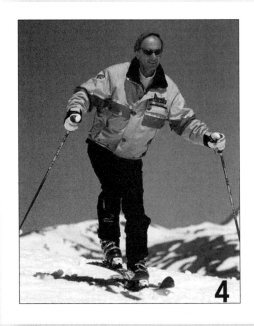

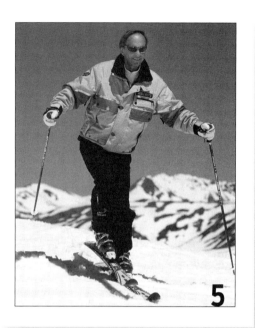
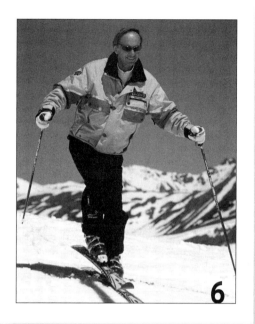

Benefits: Improves balance   **Reps:** 4 to 5

One of the best ways to prepare your body for the riggers of skiing is to force yourself to balance before it's too late—realizing what it takes to balance before you're in an irreversible position that could have been avoided. Find a low traffic area and place yourself at one side of the trail facing the opposite side. Always look up the slope before skiing or moving to be sure that the slope is clear. Point your skis slightly downhill and begin a traverse across the slope. After you start moving, pick up your uphill ski and try to balance on the lower ski the rest of the way across the slope. Practice this move in both directions. If you've never performed this exercise it may take a few attempts to learn to balance. Every good to expert skier can traverse on one ski. If you're having problems and can't seem to balance, you may need to be assessed for leg and boot alignment. Proper alignment can make a great improvement in your skiing ability and increase your fun.

Stepping

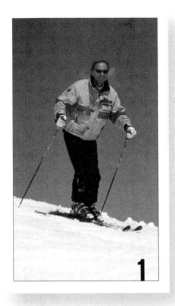

1

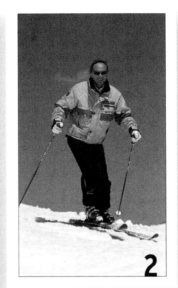

2

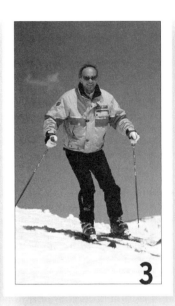

3

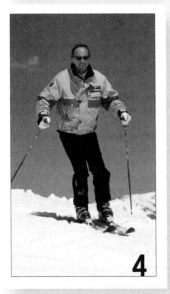

4

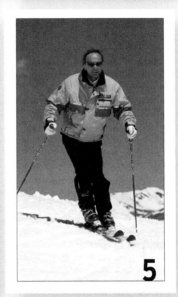

5

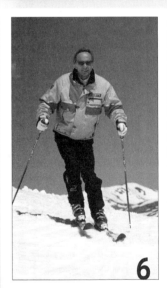

6

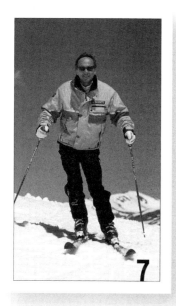 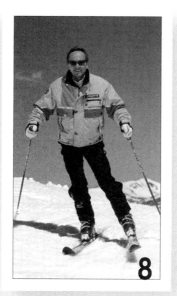 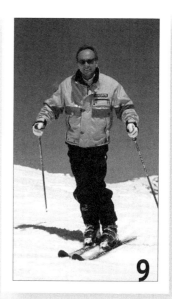

Benefits: Improves balance   Reps: 3 to 4

Stepping while moving across a slope gives you a dynamic balance warm-up. Start as you did for Balancing (page 68-69). Make sure it's safe to proceed and then point your skis slightly downhill. Push off and step the uphill ski slightly up the slope by moving the tip of the ski up the slope. Transfer your balance and weight to the stepped ski and follow up by bringing the downhill ski parallel to the stepped ski. Continue to step until you come to a stop. Now do the same exercise in the other direction. If you do this exercise three or four times in each direction you'll be ready to move down the slope with renewed confidence in your balancing ability.

Hopping

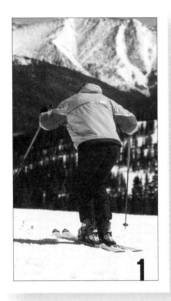
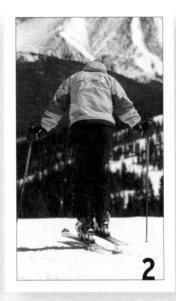
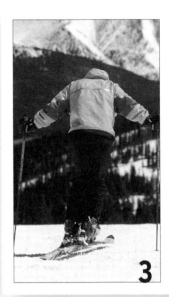

Benefits: Warms up your core   **Reps:** 2 to 3 sets of 5 to 6 hops

Hopping is a great way to get your body moving and warm up your core. It's an athletic move that requires some energy—but then so does skiing, so let's give it a try. On a very slight slope on which you're barely moving, place both poles into the snow. Use the poles to push your body off the snow while at the same time hopping into the air. While in the air change the angle of the skis to land on one set of edges. As soon as you land jump or hop again changing edges in the air to land on the other set of edges. Try to create five or six hops in a row. This exercise will absolutely prepare you for turning and gripping and you challenge yourself on the slopes.

Summary

Now you have a large and diverse set of warm-up and stretching exercises to prepare for a great day of skiing. There are probably more exercises in this book then anyone has time to do before going skiing; my suggestion is therefore to practice as many as you can at home and become familiar with the range of exercises provided. After you find those that are most beneficial to you, build a repertoire for yourself. Try to include at least one exercise for each of the important muscles groups and joint ranges of movement.

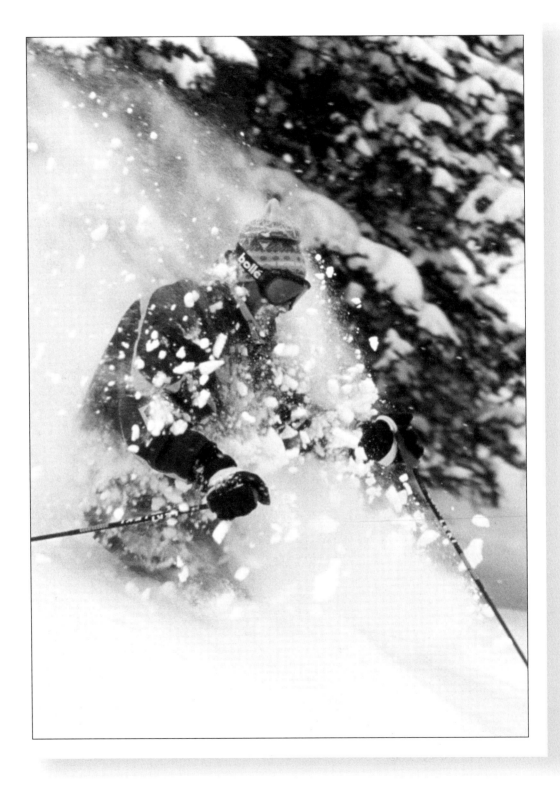

Part 3:
Year-Round
Conditioning
for Peak
Performance

SURE, SKIING IS A WINTER SPORT, BUT IF YOU WANT TO EXCEL ON THE slopes, you'd be wise to follow a year-round conditioning program. And not only to benefit your skiing performance, but also for general health benefits.

Our conditioning program includes four elements:

Cardiovascular conditioning;

Off-season strength and flexibility training;

Ski-specific exercises; and

Stretches you can perform from the time you wake up to the time you go to bed at night.

Basic Cardiovascular Training

Skiers depend on cardiovascular endurance to keep from tiring during a day of skiing. They depend on their anaerobic conditioning to reduce the fatigue and

---

burning in the muscles after short bursts on single runs. These short bursts can add up and wear you down over the period of an hour or two. A strong cardiovascular conditioning program is the foundation for full recovery after every run by the time the lift ride is over and you're on the summit again. But good cardiovascular fitness doesn't happen overnight. To keep your heart in shape for the start of the season, train regularly throughout the off-season using a heart rate-based conditioning program.

Your ability to ski longer and recover faster is dependent on your cardiovascular condition—in other words, how efficiently the heart pumps blood throughout the body and how much oxygen your lungs deliver to the blood in every beat. Cardio conditioning trains the heart and lungs to work more efficiently. Your cardiovascular condition is measured by how many beats per minute (bpm) your heart pumps during any given exercise. The fewer the beats, the more conditioned the heart.

The best way to determine your current cardio condition and create a workout that will safely improve it is to determine and monitor your target heart rate. Since skiers come at all ages and fitness levels, heart rate training is an optimal and simple way to monitor and increase the intensity of your personal workout as you get stronger. The heart is a muscle and it can be over- or under-trained. Heart rate training will keep you in the proper zone, whatever your age or fitness level.

The simplest way to monitor your heart rate is with a heart rate monitor. (Polar makes very good and inexpensive models.) Otherwise, you can find your heart rate by taking your pulse at your wrist, counting beats for 15 seconds, then multiplying the number of beats by four, for beats per minute. (To find your resting heart rate, discussed below, take your pulse for one minute on three consecutive mornings before getting out of bed, then use the average of the three rates.)

You want to train at your target heart rate, which is 70 to 80 percent of your maximum heart rate. To determine your maximum heart rate (MHR), subtract your age from 220. To determine your target heart rate (THR), multiply your MHR by .70 (for 70 percent intensity) and .80 (for 80 percent intensity). Here is an example for a 35 year old:

MHR = 220 − 35 = 185 bpm
THR = 185 x .70 = 130 bpm

THR = 185 x .80 = 148 bpm

Another target heart rate calculation, known as the heart rate reserve or Karvonen method, takes into account your resting heart rate (RHR):

[(**MHR** − **RHR**) x percent of exercise intensity] + **RHR**

Here is an example of a 35 year old's target heart rate, calculated using the Karvonen method:

MHR = 220 − 35 = 185 beats per minute
RHR = 60 beats per minute
THR = [(185 − 60) x .70] + 60 = 147 beats a minute

Whichever method you decide to use, begin with the low training range (60 to 70 percent of MHR). If you haven't done much weight-bearing or cardiovascular exercise, you'll find that your heart rate will quickly skyrocket. Stay at the lower end of intensity (60 percent of MHR) until your body adapts.

Depending on your conditioning level, you can start a cardio routine by power walking, running, or biking. Let your heart rate be your guide. If you're just beginning, start slowly for 30 minutes and maintain your heart rate at 60 percent of your maximum heart rate.

Once you can comfortably maintain your heart rate at 60 percent for 30 minutes, begin to incorporate interval training. Warm up until your heart rate reaches 60 percent and hold at that level for two minutes. Next, pick up the pace to 70 percent. Begin to slow down, and see how long it takes your heart rate to get back to 60 percent. Once your fitness level improves to the point where it takes you less than one minute, pick up your one-minute interval to an 80 percent heart rate pace. Your eventual goal is to elevate your heart rate to the 80 to 85 percent level for two minutes and then recover to a 60 percent level for a one-minute rest. A 45-minute cardio routine should include a five- to eight-minute warm-up and a five-minute cool-down with a long slow stretch afterwards.

If you're a very conditioned athlete, you can begin your training at 70 to 75 percent of your heart rate and work your way up to 90 to 95 percent two two-minute intervals.

Off-Season Training

Of course, no matter how much cardiovascular training you do, it won't necessarily keep you in shape for the very specific fitness needs involved in skiing. Because of its multifaceted demands, skiing has diverse physical requirements that can be classified into the following categories:

Explosive Power

Muscle Strength

Quickness

Although all-out explosive power is not a constant requirement for recreational skiers, there are times when you need to make an all-out power move. In most of these cases you're unaware that you're straining particular muscles, ligaments, tendons, and joints. For example, let's say you need to recover from a fall or from someone cutting in front of you. At that moment, your survival instincts automatically kick in and override your tendency to protect any unconditioned muscles needed for the recovery. In such a situation, the muscles fire quickly and powerfully—even if they're not conditioned to or haven't done so for many months or years. That's why people who ski, especially after months or years of inactivity, feel beat-up after they return to the slopes. My own personal experience confirms how much muscle activity is required the first few times on the slopes each season, despite the fact that I have been skiing my whole life. Although

Ski-Specific Muscles

The most important skiing muscles are:

Shoulders

Lower Back

Glutes (muscles around the hip and pelvis)

Legs (quads, front of thigh & hamstrings, muscles on back of thigh)

Lower legs (calf, tibialis anterior, inventors and evertors of the ankle)

I train my muscles to the best of my ability each off-season, I notice that skiing demands are still different from all preparation activities. As I grow older, I notice that staying in top physical condition is a requirement, not a luxury, if I intend to perform at the level I expect year after year.

If you're not physically prepared or conditioned for the reasonable levels of physical stress that skiing requires, you will definitely have some days of discomfort. Here are my training program recommendations and options, starting from the least consuming in time and energy to a more dedicated, higher level of preparedness.

Minimal Off-Season Fitness Program

Basic cardio program of walking or biking riding three times per week, 30 minutes per session. Work up to 40 minutes per session.

Do the introductory strength exercises (pages 80 to 86) twice per week for developing specific strength in the ski muscles.

Intermediate Off-Season Fitness Program

Bike riding, Stairmaster, or other types of similar activity three times per week, 45 minutes per session. Do both the introductory and more advanced balance and skill strength training exercises (pages 80 to 91) three times per week.

Advanced Off-Season Fitness Program

Add bike training with interval training (see *The Lance Armstrong Performance Program: Seven Weeks to the Perfect Ride*, by Lance Armstrong and Chris Carmichael) for a complete description of interval training. I also recommend, mountain biking on trails, tennis, soccer, rope jumping, or aerobics. These activities add an element of more forceful impact and require quickness, which are important in a high-level skier's preparation. High impact training is not desirable if it's overdone, but an element of impact is necessary to develop conditioning and preparation for advanced levels of skiing. You can condition the joints and muscles to absorb impact and therefore avoiding the injuries that can be caused by lack of preparation for advanced skiing conditions such as bumps, steeps, or ice.

I personally follow this Advanced Off-Season Fitness Program. I ride my bike up to four times per week for a minimum of one hour per ride. I build up to two hours a ride at least once a week. These rides consist of steep hills for at least 10 miles. I supplement my legwork with hiking and I follow a weight training workout for my upper body and abdominals.

This book offers a basic intermediate leg conditioning program that you can do in your home or office. It is not designed to guide you through an advanced weight training program. If after you've followed this program for four weeks and are motivated to take your training to the next level, you can begin a weight-training program at your local health club or gym.

Ski-Specific Indoor Exercises

Of course overall fitness is important to skiing, but some exercises are especially effective for skiers. The following exercises will challenge you and make you a better skier. In this section we'll introduce you to some equipment that will help you in your quest for ski fitness: the tipping plate and the tube.

The *tipping plate* or board is a one-footed balance and ankle muscle control training device. The balance board or plate is easy to construct; it requires one piece of wood and a single dowel. Complete construction information is on my **www.harbskisystems.com** Web site.

The *tube* is large diameter surgical tube found at most health or athletic stores. It can also be found at the PSIA.com instructors Web site. These cords commonly have a loop or handle at each end. The handle is fixed to a door jam or other anchor. The other end is fixed to the foot or ankle as needed. The tension or resistance on the cord is controlled by how far you stretch the cord before performing the exercises. There are many variations of these exercises. Slightly modifying your movement can change the muscles and benefits dramatically. For example, if you extend the leg backward and extend the leg, you're working the glutes and lower back muscles. If you move the foot back and flex at the knee you work the hamstrings. Following are the variations for the pull-back series.

The Exercises

Toe Touches

Improves: Balance

Reps: 10 with each foot

For this exercise you need a wooden block at least 4 inches wide, 2 inches high, and 12 to 20 inches long. Stand with one foot on the block and the other foot raised off the floor. The object is to touch the floor in three spots with the raised foot. The first spot is directly behind the block; the spot is to the side; and the third spot is in front of the block. To start another repetition, swing your foot in a semicircular motion back to the first spot behind the block. The movement should be continuous, without hesitation (except for the short floor touches). You may mark the spots on the floor to keep track of your range of motion. As you become more skilled you'll want to move the spots farther away from the block to increase the challenge. Go around the semicircle 10 times with each foot. You'll immediately notice the strengthening benefits of this exercise. Skiing is a balance activity, and we are frequently changing stance from one foot to the other. This exercise develops your ability to change and stabilize your body in a one-footed stance.

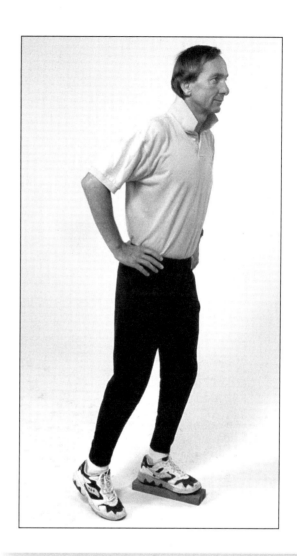

Foot Circles

Improves: Balance, body stabilization

Reps: 10 with each foot

This exercise is similar to the Toe Touches on the previous page, except that the raised foot traces a full circle on the floor (and never leaves the floor) while it moves all the way around and behind the body. This is a great balance and body stabilizing exercise. Make a circle around your block as shown in the photo. As you become more skilled, increase the diameter of the circle 1 inch at a time. Over a period of a few weeks you'll notice a big improvement in your ability to balance; this ability will transfer directly to your skiing skill.

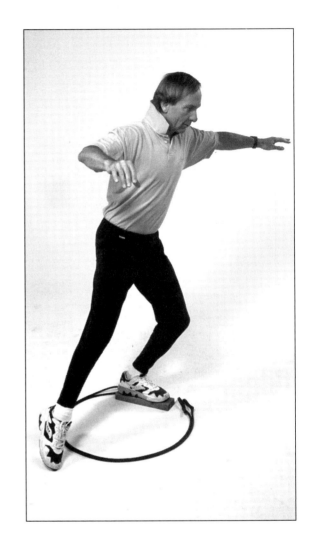

Tipping Plate*

Improves: Balance, ankle muscle control

Reps: 1 on each foot

Start in your bare feet or with sneakers on. Straddle the Tipping Plate and then center one foot on the board with your heel and your second toe on the centerline. Extend your arms (with or without poles) and lift your free foot slightly off the ground. Adjust your stance and/or foot position subtly on the board if needed. (If you always tip abruptly to one side or the other and get stuck, vary your foot position.) Balance! Repeat with the opposite foot.

* Find out how to make your own tipping plate at **www.harbskisystems.com**.

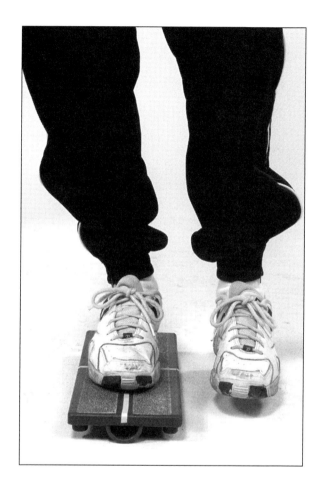

Tubing Pull Backs

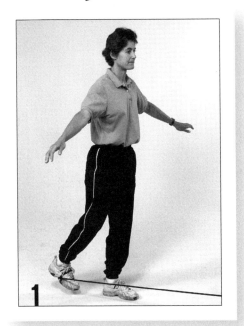

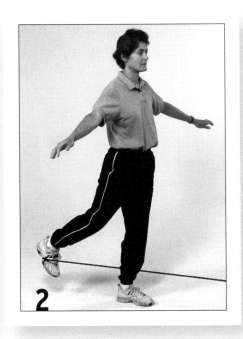

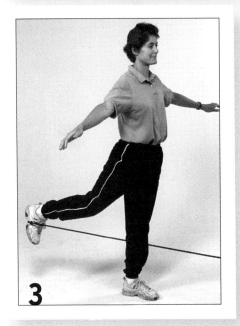

Improves: Balance; strengthens glutes, lower back, hamstrings

Reps: 3 sets of 10 on each leg

To begin, stand on one leg. This in itself is challenging! You might find that until you become more skilled with the exercise's movements the standing leg may be getting more of a workout than the flexing leg. Move the leg that has the tubing attached backward as far as you can while keeping it as straight as possible. Raise the foot off the floor as far as possible while it's behind your hips. Bring the foot back to the starting position and start again. Each pull back is considered one rep.

Behind-the-Back Leg Curls

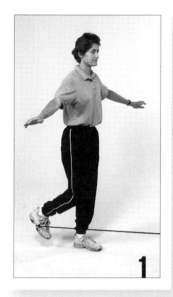 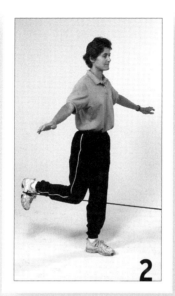 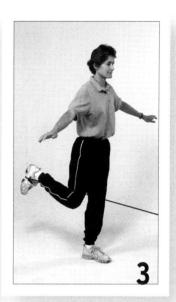

Improves: Balance, stability, overall leg muscle strength

Reps: 10 on each leg

These Leg Curls develop strength in the hamstring muscles. Start with the feet together. Flex the leg at the knee until the heel is as far behind and up as you can take it. Repeat the movement 10 times on each leg. This exercise places demands on your ability to balance and trains your overall body stability and strength, which is necessary for advanced skiing.

Leg Kicks

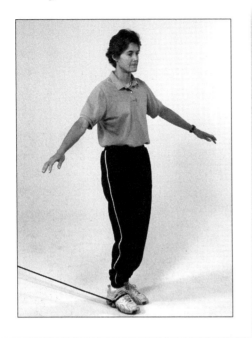 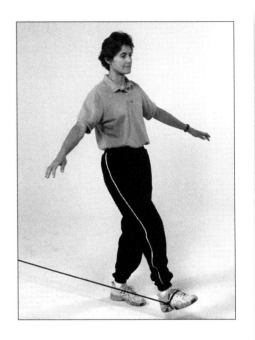

Improves: Balance, stability; strengthens hip flexor

Reps: 10 on each side

This exercise is similar to the Behind-the-Back Leg Curls on the previous pages, except that it's performed by moving the leg and foot forward. Keep your leg as straight as possible.

8 Board Exerciser and Movement Tool

The 8 Board by Grail Sports is a low-impact exercise tool that develops awareness of leg and hip movements. It's a terrific training tool for skiing in addition to tennis, golf, volleyball, and baseball.

Skiers often have difficulty developing flexibility in their hips. That flexibility is important because it allows the legs to move independently of the pelvis. Many skiers also have a hard time developing the counteracting movements that (in a ski turn) turn the hips away from the skis and allow the legs to follow the skis from a stable mid-body. The 8 Board will help you to develop and become aware of the muscles and movements that provide favorable upper and lower body movements. These movements are called *Counteracting Movements* in the book *Anyone Can Be an Expert Skier 2*.

Although all tipping movements should begin at the feet and ankles, complementary movements higher up in the kinetic chain should develop between the legs and the pelvis in the hip joints. If the mid-body doesn't move, skiers have a hard time making short, energetic turns, and that reduces their ability to ski in bumps, steeps, and powder.

Using the 8 Board everyday can also loosen the lower back muscles in a gentle, progressive way. Use it before or after skiing to help you develop a sense of leg movement in the pelvis.

The 8 Board comes with a carrying case and a complete instructional video that demonstrates how to use the 8 Board for all the sports mentioned above. For more information, check out the 8 Board Web site: **www.grailsports.com**.

The Exercises

The Slow Twister, page 88

The Spinner, page 89

The Slow Twister

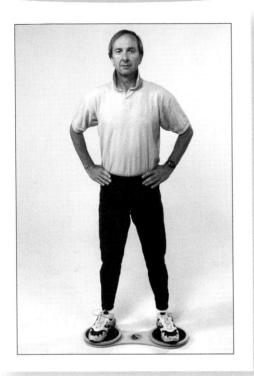 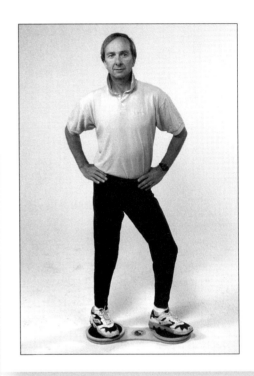

To get started with the 8 Board, put one foot in the center of each circle so that your feet are almost parallel. This exercise helps you feel your legs and hips moving from one side to the other, but in opposite directions. Move your feet in one direction and your hips in the opposite direction; try to move and twist to the end of your range of movement. Don't force it; stay in your comfort zone. Come back to the starting position and then move to the end of your range in the opposite direction. Keep moving in a fluid, continuous motion, but move slowly. You will become aware of the power you have in your hip movement to stabilize your body over your skis through the movements on 8 Board. To become more familiar with your body movements and sensations, initiate the movements in one session with your feet and then do another series of movements starting from the hips and pelvis.

The Spinner

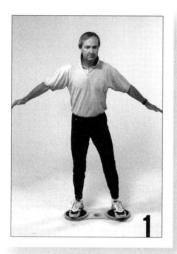 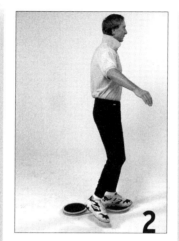 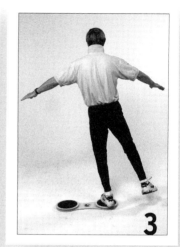

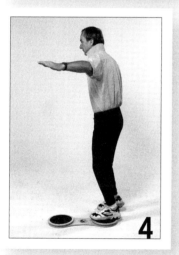

The 8 Board can be used as a balance development tool. In this exercise, you stand on one foot on one side of the 8 Board and spin in a circle. Continue to spin, making a full circle, until you've come the whole way around and are facing forward again. Then step onto the other side of the 8 Board and spin in the opposite direction. You can make up combinations of spins in any direction on one foot.

Strengthening for Serious Skiers

The following exercises can be performed anywhere, at any time—even if it's 100 degrees out and the biggest hill around is the interstate off-ramp. Use these exercises to stay fit during the off-season and when the snow starts falling again, you'll be astonished at how pain-free your first days back on the slopes will be.

Each of these exercises can be done on separate days or all on one day depending on your fitness level. If you do them all on the same day, leave at least two full days between another workout to give your legs time enough to recover.

The Exercises

Lunges, page 91

Bench Steps, page 92

Single-Leg Squats, page 93

Pro Torso Twist, page 94

Lunges

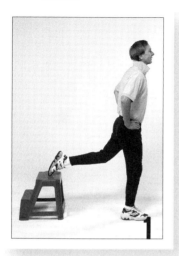
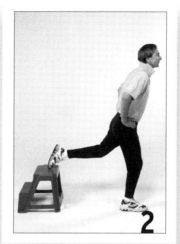
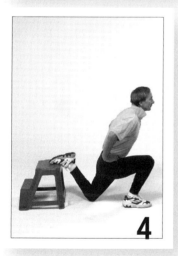
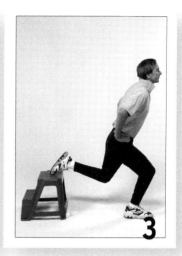

Strengthens: Upper thigh and quads

Sets/Reps: Up to 3 sets of 10 each leg

The Lunge is part of almost every serious ski-training program and it requires almost no apparatus. This exercise can be tailored to any level of fitness. If you're a beginner, do the exercise without a bench or chair; simply put one foot in front of the other, flex the front leg, and touch the knee of the back leg to the floor. If you have difficulty bending low enough, place a ball or cushion under the back knee. Once you're able to touch 10 times on each leg for three sets you can move to a more difficult level by introducing the low bench or chair for the back foot. Place the back foot on the bench and stand straight over the front leg. Flex the front leg until your thigh is parallel with the floor. For an ever tougher workout, flex until you can touch the back knee to the floor. I don't recommend you do this the first time you start your training program. It's wise to build strength gradually–for all the exercises.

Bench Steps

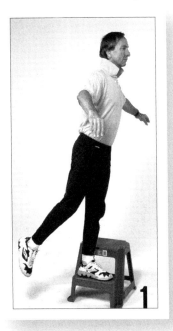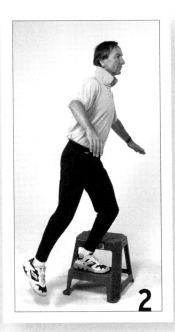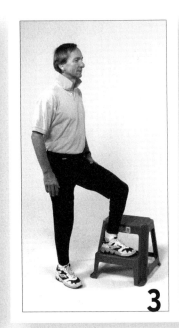

Strengthens: Upper leg

Sets/Reps: 3 sets of 10 on each leg

Notice I demonstrate the Bench Step using the lower step first. Use this exercise not only to develop your quad muscles, but also to enhance your balance. See how I step up and hold my arms to the side for balance. Just as you do when you ski, use your arms to assist your developing balance awareness. There's no secret formula to this exercise: Just put one foot on the step and use that leg to lift your body up to the new level. Stay balanced for a second or two and then step back to the floor with the back foot. Be careful not to assist the step with the foot that's on the floor, because the idea is to use the muscles on the upper leg to lift your body. Do 10 lifts on each leg before switching. Build up to three sets on each leg before moving to a higher bench. This may take two to three weeks.

Single-Leg Squats

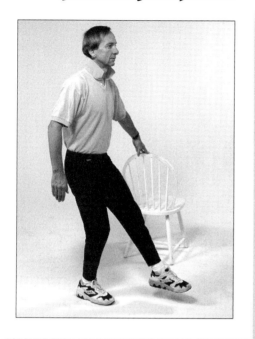 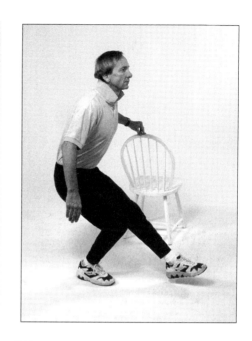

Strengthens: Quads

Sets/Reps: 3 sets of 10 on each leg

These squats are an advanced strength training exercise, especially if you lower your hips until your thigh is parallel to the floor. At first, you should use the chair to assist your balance and strength. And remember that there's no need to go low into flexion on your first go-round. Flex low enough so you can feel the top and front of your leg muscles tensing. Hold the other leg out front and keep it straight. Try to work up to 3 sets of 10 repetitions on each leg.

Pro Torso Twist

Strengthens: Lower back and abs

Reps: 8 to 12 on each side

This exercise is quite similar to the Torso Twists on pages 26 and 27, but this is a more advanced version for serious athletes who want to increase lower back and ab strength and flexibility. Lie on the floor with your legs extended and nearly perpendicular to the floor. Spread your arms to the side for stability and to keep your lower back on the floor. You may have to push your arms against the floor to keep the upper body from moving. Move your legs to one side until the outside leg touches the floor. Bring the legs back to the starting position and then move them to the other side.

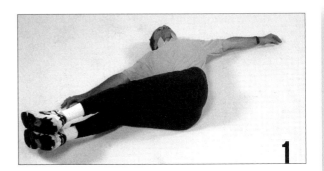

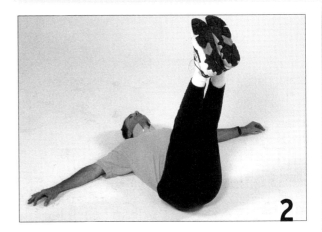

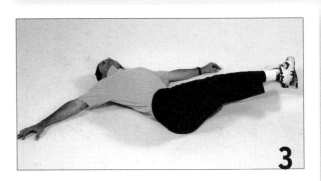

Stretching Throughout the Day

You may be saying, "The Ski Flex program is great, but how am I going to stretch during the week? I hardly have time to eat breakfast and kiss the family good-bye. I just don't have time for a flexibility program."

This is the beauty of Ski Flex. You can practice your flexibility routine anywhere—at home, in the car, or at the office. Just do a few minutes at a time and you'll achieve long-term results. Here's how you can incorporate these stretches into your daily life.

In Bed

Do these stretches before you get out of bed in the morning and your back will love you. Bring one knee to your chest, hold for 10 seconds, and then alternate knees. Next, bring both knees to your chest and hold for 10 seconds. Fold your knees over to one side, then the other, holding for 10 seconds each. Be sure to keep your shoulders flat on the bed. As your flexibility increases, move smoothly from one position to the next. These stretches will warm up, stretch, and prepare your back and spine for the day!

Rise and Shine!

Give yourself a big hug, stretching your upper- and mid-back. Hold one arm across your chest and hug it toward you with the opposite hand. Alternate arms, stretching the shoulder muscles.

From either a seated or standing position, interlace your fingers and lift your hands over your head, pushing your palms away from you. This stretches your forearms, shoulders, and rib cage. This exercise can be increased by gently leaning over to one side, stretching your waist. Be sure to keep your abdominal muscles tight while doing this stretch.

Time to Shower

A nice hot shower offers an excellent opportunity to warm up and stretch. Start by letting the hot water hit the back of your neck, relaxing your upper back and neck muscles. Slowly do half circles, letting your chin roll from one shoulder to the other. Repeat approximately six times.

Now that your back is warmed up, do a few upper body rotations. Let the water run down your upper- and mid-back. Hold each stretch for 10 seconds. Reach forward with both hands, roll your shoulders forward, and feel the stretch in your back. Now clasp your hands behind you and stick out your chest like a rooster crowing. Turn and face the water, letting it warm your chest muscles. You have just had a great upper-body stretch and in no time. Shower everyday, stretch everyday—see the difference it makes!

Toweling Off

Grab a towel at both ends, bringing one hand over your head and one behind your back. Reverse the motion and rotate your hands. This is a wonderful way to stretch your rotator cuffs and keep your shoulders healthy.

Stand with one foot forward, bending your rear knee and keeping your front leg straight while you towel off. To increase this stretch, wrap the towel around your forward foot and gently pull toward you. This exercise increases the strength and flexibility of your calves and Achilles tendons.

Reading the Paper

You do it every morning! Take this time to also strengthen your hands and fore-arms. After reading a section of the paper, take a sheet in one hand and slowly crumble it into a tight ball. This is a lot harder than it seems. Try getting up to four sheets per hand.

Getting Dressed

Putting on a shirt is something we do everyday and it can be a great stretch for our shoulders, rib cage, and arms. As you put one arm through your shirt, reach as far as you can toward the sky, and repeat with the opposite arm.

Putting on Socks and Shoes

While seated, cross one ankle over the opposite knee and feel the stretch in the back of your legs and butt as you lean over to put on your sock.

Reverse leg position and put on the other sock. Then slip on your shoes. Go down on one knee as you tie your shoe, stretching the front of your hip and your back leg.

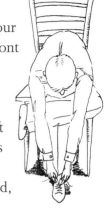

Sitting in the Car, Waiting for It to Warm Up

Keep your right hand on the steering wheel and reach your left hand across your body to the back of your seat. This really opens up your back and shoulders. Repeat on the opposite side.

Interlace both hands behind your head and reach backward, stretching both your chest and back.

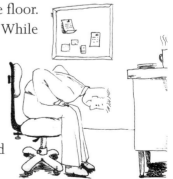

At the Office

For many us, sitting at the office all day can make us tight and often tense. Sitting with our legs crossed for hours at a time while hunched over a desk does nothing to promote flexibility. But by taking just a few minutes a day, you can easily increase your well-being and flexibility. There's an old Italian saying, *Chi va piano va sano e lontano*. It means, "He who goes slowly, goes safely and far."

Sit with your left ankle over your right knee. Keeping your spine straight, place your right hand on your left knee, and turn your torso to your left. While in the same position, turn your torso to the right by placing your left hand on the outside of your right thigh.

This is a great spine stretch! Continue by placing both hands on your thighs and gently lower your chest toward your knees, stretching your butt, back, and thighs. Reverse feet position and repeat.

Sit with your feet flat on the floor and slowly drop your head between your knees, letting your hands fall to the floor. You will feel this stretch in your lower back and butt. While in this stretch position, remember to breathe deeply into your lower back, filling your lungs and slowly letting tension release with each exhale.

Grab both sides of the doorway with your hands at shoulder level. Walk forward until you feel the stretch in your arms. This exercise is great for your chest and shoulder muscles.

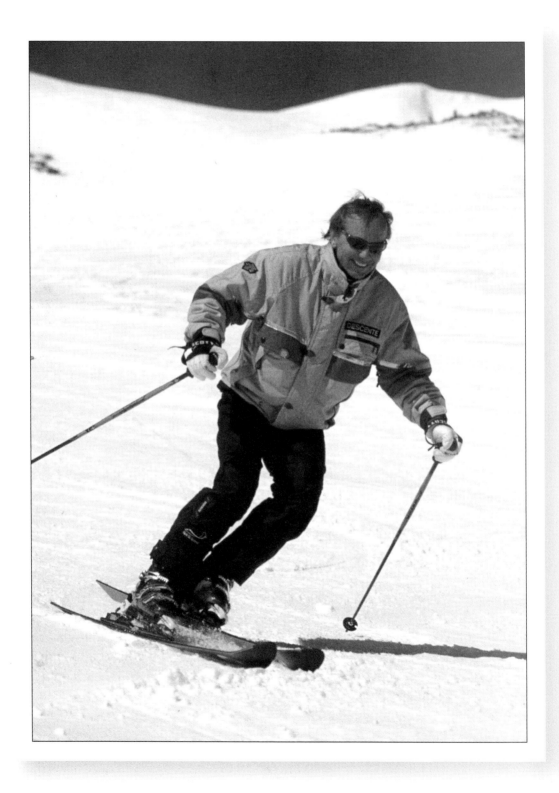

Part 4:

A Final Note

SKI FLEX WAS DEVELOPED OUT OF NECESSITY. AFTER LISTENING TO SKIERS spend every Monday complaining about muscle weakness and soreness after skiing a couple of hours over the weekend, we encouraged everyone to follow this program.

The response we always got was, "Of course I work out and stretch. Everyone stretches before they hit the slopes. That's nothing new. Everyone knows the benefits of training and how it affects your performance." But if they were preparing properly, why were they always so banged up and sore? So we asked them how they stretched. The response was always the same. "Oh, well, I…uh, you know, uh…do some of these and then I bend this way, and…uh, you know, loosen up."

It was pretty obvious that they didn't have a handle on what they were doing, and that they probably picked up most of what they did from what they saw other skiers doing in the lodge. Skiers know skiing, not stretching. It was apparent that they had no systematic approach to stretching that they could follow in a systematic way.

We developed Ski Flex so skiers could understand and perform stretches and warm-ups in a simple and clear manner. We also included some basic strengthening exercises and routines, because unless you begin to increase overall strength there will be some limitations to your skiing development. Balance is the most important part of learning to ski. Increase your ability to balance and you'll increase your skiing enjoyment. Sometimes we lose balance due to lack of muscle tone or an imbalance in the co-contracting muscle groups around joints. Following the balancing routines in this book will help you become aware of your balancing ability.

Ski Flex not only improves your skiing, but it also leads to increased body awareness and well-being. You can achieve wonderful results, so what are you waiting for? When it comes to stretching, there's never an excuse not to do something.

In Health and Fitness,
Paul Frediani and *Harald Harb*

Meet the Authors

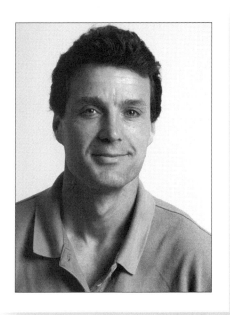

Paul Frediani

Paul, who is an educator for the American Council of Exercise, became interested in fitness when he was 12 years old, surfing the chilly waters in San Francisco. His interest led him to compete in open ocean swims, long-distance running, and triathlons. He won the San Francisco Golden Gloves and the Pacific Coast Diamond Belt Light-Heavy Weight Boxing Championships. Paul is certified by the American Exercise College of Sports Medicine and is a medical exercise specialist. He is affiliated with Equinox Gyms in New York City.

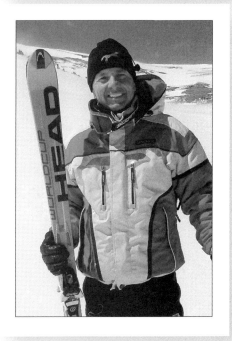

Harald Harb

Born in Austria, Harald moved to Canada at an early age and began to ski, winning his first regional race in Quebec's Laurentian Mountains at age eight. He raced in his first World Cup race at 18 with the Canadian National Ski Team and was later Overall Pro Ski Champion on the U.S. regional circuit. He has directed and coached programs that have produced some of the USA's most successful National Team members and Olympic medallists. He spent four years on the U.S. National Demonstration Team. Among his many ski education systems are the Primary Movements Teaching System™ (PMTS) and the Harb Skier Alignment System™. Harald is also a contributor to Skiing Magazine.

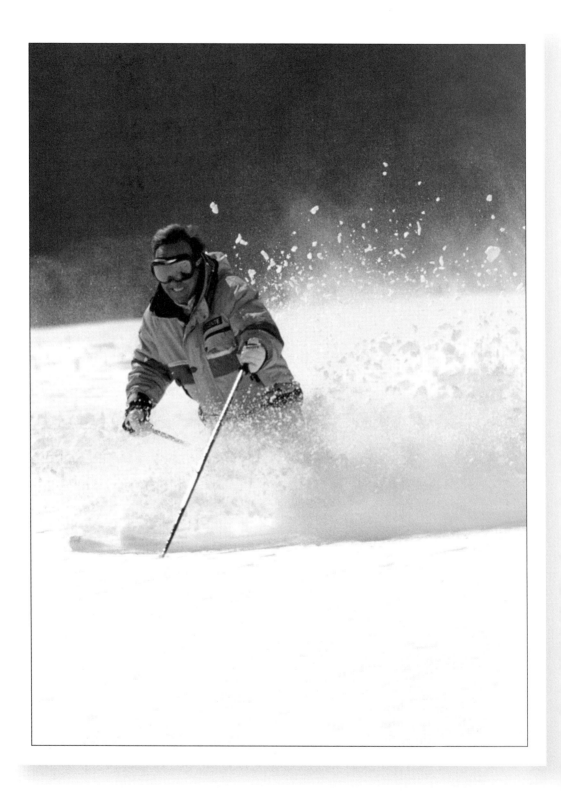

Ski with
Harald Harb

Here's your chance to ski with Harald Harb and his hand-selected and personally trained staff.

This is a ski experience you will never forget—it could change your skiing for life. Harald Harb and Diana Rogers are the authors and producers of the Anyone Can be an Expert Skier book and video series. Their company, Harb Ski Systems, offers camps and individual lessons using the techniques described in their books and videos for skiers of all levels and abilities.

Harald invented the **PMTS Direct Parallel**® system, which has caught the imagination of skiers and ski instructors all over the USA. Harald is also a pioneer in the art of alignment, foot bed design, and boot fitting. All Harb Ski Systems' Green/Blue and Blue/Dark Blue camps include indoor and on-snow alignment evaluations. The All-Mountain and Race camps include an on-snow evaluation, while indoor evaluations can be scheduled individually outside of camp hours.

For more information about the Harb Ski Systems camps— including enrollment details, schedules, and prices—visit the Harb Ski Systems Web site: www.harbskisystems.com or call 303-567-4663.

Announcing a breakthrough in the science of Expert Skiing...

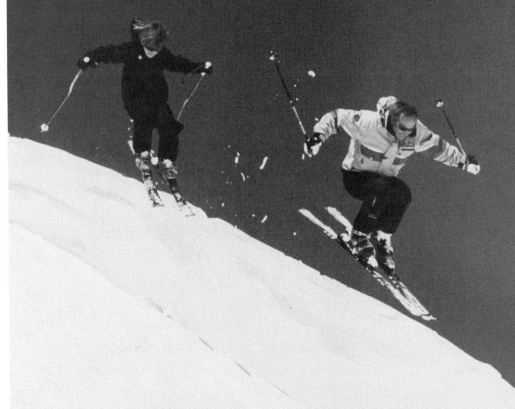

Anyone Can Be An EXPERT SKIER

BOOK & VIDEO SERIES

Release the expert skier within you!

Join skiing pioneer Harald Harb as he teaches you with his revolutionary PMTS Direct Parallel method of ski instruction. The **Anyone Can Be An Expert Skier** book and video series is the most innovative and effective teaching system ever created! You'll learn to ski expert terrain with more ease and less effort than you thought possible.

Harald Harb has spent a lifetime perfecting the PMTS Direct Parallel method. It has been used in over 100,000 lessons worldwide. Skiers and instructors alike agree that it works faster and better than any other system available. The **Anyone Can Be An Expert Skier** series will show you how to master the mountain in record time!

The **Anyone Can Be An Expert Skier** series teaches you techniques of expert skiing that anyone can learn and shows you how to choose the proper boots and skis to maximize your skiing power. The door to enjoyable, exhilarating skiing is finally open for you!

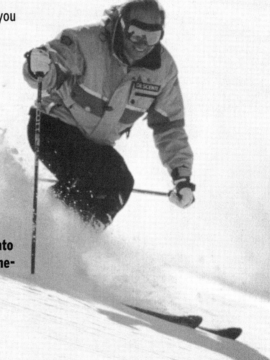

Anyone Can Be An Expert Skier

books contain over 200 photos and unique photomontages. Plus, bonus tear-out "Pocket Instructor" cards allow you to learn on the slopes.

"I have learned a lot from Harald Harb. His insights into the multiple makeup of expert skiing–equipment, biomechanics, and functional primary movements–are vital, accurate, and above all, immediately useful."

Anyone Can Be An Expert Skier 1
The New Way to Ski

Harald Harb enthusiastically offers a step-by-step, easy-to-follow process that will improve your skiing no matter what your ability level. With Harb's revolutionary PMTS Direct Parallel method, you will be on the fast track to all-mountain expert skiing! What's more, you'll learn to recognize, correct and avoid the dead-end movements that keep you from achieving your skiing potential.

Easy-to-understand and impressively complete, this book is a "must have" for skiers everywhere. Quite simply, it is regarded as the foremost authoritative guide to the art of carving with shaped skis.

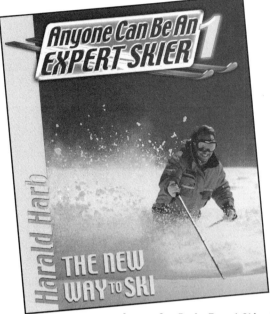

Anyone Can Be An Expert Skier 1-
The New Way to Ski
Book (ISBN 1-57826-073-6) .$19.95
Video (ISBN 1-57826-082-5) $24.95

Anyone Can Be An Expert Skier 2
Powder, Bumps, and Carving

Revealed here for the first time: the secrets of the Biomechanical Advantage—a proven technique used by hundreds of pro skiers to achieve winning performance!

In this book and video, you'll learn how to handle challenging terrains and conditions with ease. Moguls, powder and crud, steeps—there will be no limit to your skiing horizons! The special section on advanced carving techniques will perfect your skiing style—giving you precision and control like never before.

Anyone Can Be An Expert Skier 2 is your ideal solution for all mountain conditions. You will discover the techniques that have helped thousands of skiers reach the pinnacle of expert status. Guaranteed!

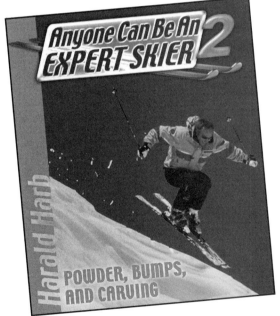

Anyone Can Be An Expert Skier 2
Powder, Bumps, and Carving
Book (ISBN 1-57826-074-4) .$19.95
Video (ISBN 1-57826-083-3) $24.95

Net Flex:
10 Minutes a Day to Better Tennis

The Secret to a Better Tennis Game is Simple—Flexibility.

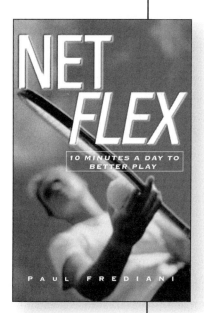

Improve your game, increase your power, speed and agility in just 10 minutes each day!

Whether you're a weekend player or a semi-pro, you can now discover the benefits of flexibility long-enjoyed by the world's top-seeded players. **Net Flex** is a simple, easy-to-follow program that is specifically designed to prepare and warm up the muscles used in tennis.

Here are just some of the ways **Net Flex** will give you an advantage on the court:

- **MONSTER SERVES! Net Flex** will increase your power and range of motion.
- **BIGGER BACKHAND! Net Flex** will teach you to use muscle memory to better your mechanics.
- **BETTER BASELINE! Net Flex** will increase your agility to play a better baseline...and a better net.

Developed by one of America's leading fitness advisors, the **Net Flex** program can be done almost everywhere—in your office, at the clubhouse, at home or on the court.

Net Flex by Paul Frediani, ACSM
Just $9.95 at bookstores everywhere
(if you don't see it, ask for it) or call 1-800-906-1234.

For more exciting books on fitness and sports,
visit our website www.healthylivingbooks.com.
Sign up today for our FREE monthly e-mail newsletter.

ISBN 1-57826-077-9

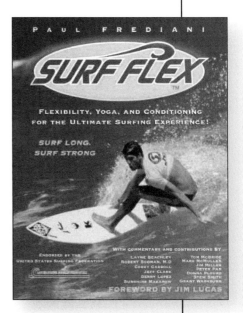

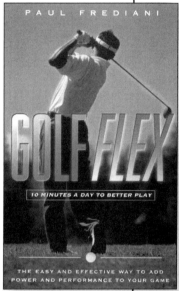
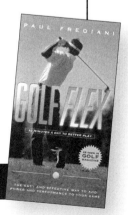